Smoking, Personality, and Stress

H.J. Eysenck

Smoking, Personality, and Stress

Psychosocial Factors in the Prevention of Cancer and Coronary Heart Disease

With 10 Illustrations

Springer-Verlag
New York Berlin Heidelberg London
Paris Tokyo Hong Kong Barcelona

H.J. Eysenck, Ph.D.
Institute of Psychiatry
University of London
London, SE5 8AF England

Library of Congress Cataloging-in-Publication Data
Eysenck, H.J. (Hans Jürgen), 1916–
    Smoking, personality, and stress: psychosocial factors in the prevention of cancer and
    coronary heart disease / Hans J. Eysenck.
        p.   cm.
    Includes bibliographical references.
    ISBN 0-387-97493-8 (alk. paper). — ISBN 3-540-97493-8 (alk.
paper)
        1. Cancer—Epidemiology   2. Smoking—Health aspects.   3. Coronary
    heart disease—Epidemiology   4. Stress (Psychology).   I. Title.
        [DNLM: 1. Coronary Disease—prevention & control.   2. Neoplasms—
    prevention & control.   3. Personality.   4. Smoking—adverse
    effects.   5. Smoking—psychology.   6. Stress, Psychological.   QV
    137 E985s]
    RA645.C3E98   1991
    616.1′205—dc20
    DNLM/DLC
    for Library of Congress   90-10443

Printed on acid-free paper.

Typeset by Best-set Typesetting, Ltd., Chai Wan, Hong Kong.
Printed and bound by R.R. Donnelley & Sons, Harrisonburg, Virginia.
Printed in the United States of America.

9 8 7 6 5 4 3 2 1

ISBN 0-387-97493-8 Springer-Verlag New York Berlin Heidelberg
ISBN 3-540-97493-8 Springer-Verlag Berlin Heidelberg New York

"There are two classes of disease—bodily and mental. Each arises from the other. Neither is perceived to exist without the other. Mental disorders arise from physical ones, and likewise physical disorders arise from mental ones."

—Mahabharata: *Santi Parva*, XVII 8–9

Preface

It is often suggested that the incidence of cancer and coronary heart disease (CHD) could be much reduced or even eliminated if only people ceased to smoke cigarettes and reduced their cholesterol level through appropriate eating. The evidence suggests that such views are simplistic and unrealistic and that cancer and CHD are the product of many risk factors acting synergistically. Psychosocial factors (stress, personality) are some six times as predictive as smoking, cholesterol level, and blood pressure and also have proved to be much more accessible to prophylactic treatment. There is no such evidence concerning quitting smoking, which seems to have only minimal effects on future health. There is no doubt that smoking is one of many risk factors, which include stress, personality, and genetic predisposition, but its effects, acting by itself, have been exaggerated. This book suggests a more realistic appraisal of a very complex chain of events, incorporating many diverse factors, and points to appropriate action to prevent cancer and CHD.

Contents

1
Introduction: Debate Concerning the Effects of Smoking on Health

Laymen and medical professionals alike often ask questions regarding the cause of cancer and coronary heart disease (CHD), the two major killers in present-day civilization, expecting a simple answer like "smoking causes cancer and coronary heart disease." Or cholesterol, produced by an unwise diet, may be blamed. It need hardly be argued that to look for single causes for complex phenomena is not a meaningful occupation, particularly when it is obvious that smoking (or the failure to use polyunsaturated fats) is neither a sufficient nor a necessary cause of lung cancer and the other diseases associated with smoking. Out of 10 heavy smokers, only one will die of lung cancer; hence, clearly, smoking is not a *sufficient* cause; there must be many other factors that, possibly in conjunction with smoking, produce a final result of death from lung cancer. Similarly, smoking is not a *necessary* cause; at least 1 in 10 people who die of lung cancer is a non-smoker, and among the Mongoloid races, the figure drops to about 1 in 2 (Eysenck, 1965, 1986). Likewise, many people who die of CHD are non-smokers. Thus, there clearly is a highly complex net of causal factors, and a stress on only one of these is scientifically meaningless, particularly if their interaction is synergistic (multiplicative).

Early reports (U.S. Surgeon General, 1979; Royal College of Physics, 1991) of a statistical association between cigarette smoking and cancer and CHD led to extrapolations from these statistical data to possible savings of lives if people were to quit smoking or never to smoke. According to reports of the U.S. Surgeon General (1982), cancer was responsible for approximately 412,000 deaths annually in the United States; the report estimated that in 1982, 430,000 deaths would be due to cancer: 233,000 among men and 197,000 among women. The report claimed that 22% to 38% of these deaths "can be attributed to smoking, and therefore are, potentially, avoidable" if smoking did not exist in human behavior. The report clearly suggests a *causal* interpretation of the *statistical* association between smoking and lung and other cancers, and it is this interpretation of the data that many experts have criticized (e.g., Berkson, 1958; Berkson & Elveback, 1960; Burch, 1976, 1978, 1983, 1986; Eysenck 1986; Fisher,

1959; Katz, 1969; Mainland & Herrera, 1956; Oeser, 1979; Seltzer, 1989; Sterling, 1973, 1977; Yerushalmy, 1966; and many others). The purpose of this book is to examine the claims made by the supporters of this "orthodox" view in light of the criticisms made by leading statisticians, epidemiologists, and oncologists, and to attempt to decide to what extent the claims made for this view are scientifically acceptable. In a later chapter, an attempt will also be made to consider facts and data not accomodated by the "orthodox" view, such as the relationship between personality and cancer and between stress and cancer. I will also examine some alternative theories. Last, I will consider similar data in relation to CHD, which is also often claimed to be statistically and causally related to smoking. The evidence here has been equally subject to criticism, and I will review this in some detail. Here, too, alternative theories may explain many of the facts not covered by the orthodox view.

How Many Deaths Are Due to Smoking?

The theory that smoking plays a *causal* role in the etiology of cancer, CHD, and various other disorders has given rise to speculation, as already mentioned, about the number of lives that could be saved if smoking could be prevented. Burch (1978) quotes studies by Higginson and Doll, claiming that we should be able to reduce the incidence of cancer "by at least 80%–90%" if cigarette smoking could be eliminated, and the U.S. Surgeon General's report (1982) states that "it is estimated that 85% of lung cancer cases are due to cigarette smoking," and that consequently "85% of lung cancer mortalities could have been avoided if individuals never took up smoking." In a speech on January 11, 1978, the Secretary of the Department of Health, Education and Welfare in the United States, Joseph Califano, stated that in 1977, smoking caused 220,000 deaths from heart disease, 78,000 from lung cancer, and 22,000 from other cancers, including bladder cancer, for a total of 320,000 deaths. One month later, Secretary Califano attributed to cigarette smoking 15,000 deaths from chronic bronchitis and emphysema, 125,000 from heart disease, and 100,000 from cancer, and stated the total to be "more than 320,000." No source was given for any of these figures, and no explanation given for why chronic bronchitis and emphysema were included in the February total but not in the January one. He also failed to explain how his estimate of smoking accounts for 40% of all cancer deaths yearly, double that suggested by the American Cancer Society.

In a similar vein, Dr. David Owen, former Minister of Health and Social Services in the United Kingdom, stated that 50,000 deaths in the United Kingdom were due to smoking and could have been prevented by people stopping smoking.

Similar sums have been done in Europe. Thus, a recent report by Roos, Vernet, and Abelin (1989) gives rather imaginary figures for the number of deaths caused by smoking in different Swiss cantons, basing their conclusions on the hypothesis that lung cancer is caused to an extent of 90% in males and 50% in females by cigarette smoking and that bronchitis and emphysema are so caused in 75% and 60% of all cases in males and females, respectively. Atteslander (1989) has cogently criticized this report on grounds that also apply to many other similar publications—lack of care in handling official statistics, confusion of definitions, and eccentric calculating methods; difficulties in establishing cause–effect relationship; and many others.

As others have done before, Abelin (1988) and the World Health Organization (1988) draw the conclusion that what is needed is a campaign to eradicate smoking, assuming that, in the words of Vecchia, Levi, and Gutzwiller (1987), smoking is "une épidemie évitable."

Of particular interest in this connection is *The Big Kill*, a 15-volume document launched by The Health Education Council jointly with the British Medical Association, one volume issued for each of the 15 regional health authorities in England and Wales (Roberts & Graveling, 1986). According to this publication, smoking annually kills 77,774 people (55,107 men and 22,667 women in England and Wales, from heart disease, lung cancer, bronchitis and emphysema. And because of their smoking, some 108,218 people are hospitalized each year with these diseases. As Burch (1986) comments: "The biologically ignorant but numerate reader will be forgiven for concluding that epidemiology is not only a rigorous science but an incredibly accurate one, with an implied error in mortality estimates of less than 1 part in 77,774" (p. 956).

The latest report of the U.S. Surgeon General (1989) continues this type of argumentation. The Surgeon General stated that "smoking will continue as the leading cause of preventable, premature death for many years to come. . . . As a result of decisions to quit smoking or not to start, an estimated 789,000 smoking-related deaths were avoided or postponed between 1964 and 1985. Furthermore, these decisions will result in the avoidance or postponement of an estimated 2.1 million smoking-related deaths between 1986 and the year 2000" (p. IV). Can this really be true?

Burch (1986) raises two questions. The first relates to the recording and certification of the cause of death. To show the utter unreliability of such figures, he quotes a study by Heasman and Lipworth (1966), who surveyed reports from 75 hospitals, comparing the clinicians' diagnoses of the cause of death with the pathologist's necropsy report. For example, clinicians diagnosed 338 cases of lung cancer, whereas pathologists discovered 417 cases post mortem. In only 227 instances, however, was agreement obtained! If the pathologist's report were correct, then 111, or 33% of the clinicians' diagnoses, were false-positive, while 190 genuine cases (46%) of lung cancer were missed. This is terrifying error rate when one considers that all the published estimates of death from smoking are based on such worthless figures. The issue of unreliability of death certificates is so vital that I will return to it in some detail later.

Burch's (1986) second point is equally important. It relates to the question of how a statistical association between smoking and disease is converted into a causal estimate of the proportion of deaths that are due to smoking. As the Royal College of Physicians (1971) admits. "It is not possible to give a precise estimate of the proportion of these excessive deaths among smokers which are caused by smoking. There can be little doubt that at least half the estimated 31,000 excess deaths among male smokers, aged 35–64, in the United Kingdom, were due to smoking." As Burch comments: "This passage shows a recognition by the Royal College that not all of the association between smoking and mortality is necessarily causal. However, no procedure is described whereby an objective estimate of the magnitude of the causal contribution might be derived and the choice "at least half" would seem to be arbitrary" (p. 956). Thus, the unreliability of the estimates of cause of death is multiplied by the arbitrariness of causal attribution; why one-half rather than one-quarter?

The Royal College makes additional arbitrary attribution estimates, "It should not be unreasonable to attribute to cigarette-smoking 90% of the deaths from lung cancer, 75% from chronic bronchitis and 25% of those from coronary heart disease." For women, the report acknowledges the greater difficulty of precise attribution but continues undaunted to say, "It can reasonably be assumed that at least 40% of the deaths from lung cancer, 60% of those from bronchitis, and 20% of those from coronary heart disease in women aged 35–64 may well be due to cigarette smoking." The sophisticated reader will be aware that expressions like "would not be unreasonable," "may well be due to," and "it can reasonably be assumed that," have no scientific standing or meaning; they refer simply to guesses that can easily be doubled or halved. Thus, *The Big Kill* raises the percentage of deaths from cigarette smoking for lung cancer in women from 40% (Royal Society) to 80%, without batting an eyelid. Such estimates are meaningless, even if the figures for the *statistical association* between smoking and disease could be accepted. As I shall demonstrate, that is by no means so; these figures are based on studies characterized by a combination of poor methodology and faulty reasoning.

Burch summarized his conclusions from these considerations as follows:

We have to bear in mind that the reports of the Royal College of Physicians and of the U.S. Surgeon-General were prepared by committees with a predominantly medical background and outlook. Their primary concern, therefore, is likely to have been with the avoidance of unnecessary suffering and premature death. No one can quarrel with these aims and the good intentions permeating the reports. The process of reaching sound conclusions about causation is, however, more of a scientific than a medical task. Medical skills are required, of course, to reach an accurate diagnosis of the cause of death and a proper appreciation of limitations in the evidence, but analysis of the resulting statistics calls for familiarity and dexterity with scientific logic. The two skills are not incompatible but they are not always combined in the same person. We may note that Feinstein, (1988), himself both a distinguished clinical epidemiologist and an expert medical statistician, protests that a "licensed" epidemiologist " . . . can obtain and manipulate the data in diverse ways that are sanctioned not by the delineated standards of science, but by the traditional practice of epidemiologists." (Burch, 1986, p. 957)

What are these "traditional practices?" The U.S. Surgeon General reproduces in his 1982 Report a passage from the first report about smoking and health by the Surgeon General, published in 1964. It encapsulates a methodology cum philosophy that enjoys a wide support among epidemiologists:

The causal significance of an association is a matter of judgment which goes beyond any statement of statistical probability. To judge or evaluate the causal significance of the association between an attribute or agent and the disease, or the effect upon health, a number of criteria must be utilized, no one of which is an all-sufficient basis for judgment. These criteria include: (a) the consistency of the association; (b) the strength of the association; (c) the specificity of the association; (d) the temporal relationship of the association, and (e) the coherence of the association."

The inadequacy of these poorly defined criteria and the dubious manner of their application to the association between smoking and lung cancer have been discussed at length elsewhere (Burch, 1983). With reference to the Surgeon General's (1982) point c, Brownlee (1965) commented, "The way it [the 1964 Report] claims the facts are in comformity with the criterion is to flatly ignore the facts" (p. 724). That comment remains applicable not only to c but to all five criteria. Subjective judgment, on which the U.S. Surgeon General places repeated emphasis, should play as limited a role as possible in epidemiology as in other sciences. How do we distinguish between judgment and prejudice? "Scientific analysis aims to replace subjective judgment by the objective testing of hypotheses" (Burch, 1986, p. 957).

With these conclusions it is difficult to find fault, and the rest of this book is devoted to a consideration of the evidence and the conclusions that may justifiably be drawn from this evidence.

There is one additional point to be considered in connection with the statement by the Royal College of Physicians and the U.S. Surgeon General concerning the number of deaths that are directly due to smoking. The statement quoted about the "excess deaths among smokers which are caused by smoking" is not really intelligible without being related to a precise model of causation. What precisely does it mean to say that 40% (or 80%!) of deaths from lung cancer in women are due to cigarette smoking? Several models might serve to mediate such interaction between smoking and disease.

The first model asserts that out of the 10 deaths from lung cancer in women, 4 (or 8) are directly and solely due to smoking. This simple-minded model hardly can be intended to be taken seriously, but the arguments advanced by the U.S. Surgeon General and the Royal College of Physicians often seem to assume its correctness. The notion that risk factors other than smoking play absolutely no part in these deaths conflicts with all we know about smoking and its many connections with other risk factors (drinking, stress, life-style etc.) and is quite untenable.

A second model asserts that there are many risk factors for lung cancer (or CHD, or whatever disease is linked with smoking) and that, in every sufferer from lung cancer, 40% (or 80%) of these risk factors are constituted by cigarette smoking. This scenario also is unrealistic; it is simply not reasonable to assume that the proportion of all risk factors contributing to disease is identical for all sufferers, and there is solid evidence to contradict it, as will be shown in later chapters. This model, too, often seem to be asumed by writers on the subject.

A third model asserts that risk factors are unevenly spread among sufferers, so that the percentages mentioned apply only on average but not in any particular case. Thus, for a smoker who has been in touch with asbestos, the percentage of risk that is due to smoking might be only 10%, while for someone else not associated with any other risk factor, the percentage might be 100%. This model seems more realistic, but of course, it suffers from the fact that there is no known method of calculating the importance of risk factors for individuals. The model also makes the unlikely assumption that risk factors act in a simple additive fashion; as demonstrated in the following discussion, the evidence strongly opposes such a view.

Finally, the fourth model seems to be more in accord with the facts than any of the preceding models. It asserts that smoking linked diseases are caused by multiple risk factors combining synergistically, that is, the interaction is multiplicative rather than additive. The evidence for this model will be discussed in a later section, but some of the papers supporting this view follow: Eysenck, 1988b; Grossarth-Maticek, 1980b, 1989; Grossarth-Maticek, Eysenck and Vetter, 1988; and Grossarth-Maticek, Vetter, and Frentzel-Beyme, 1988. The evidence suggests very strongly that smoking by itself has *little* effect on cancer or CHD; in samples free from other risk factors, smoking hardly correlates at all with these diseases. It is only in combination with other risk factors (in particular psychosocial ones) that smoking shows statistical associations with these disease (e.g. Grossarth-Maticek, 1980 b; Grosssarth-Maticek, Eysenck, Vetter, 1988). Whether these statistical associations can be interpreted in a *causal* manner is still an unsolved question.

Dembrowski (1984) reaches similar conclusions:

The findings reviewed clearly indicate that there are very complex relationships present involving classic risk factors, stress, personality attributes, consummatory behaviors, and physiologic reactivity. Moreover, the observation that many consummatory behaviors covary, e.g. cigarette smoking, caffeine, alcohol, etc., and that each can affect cardiovascular reactions to stress, makes it clear that sorting out individual and interactive effects is a complex challenge for future research. Even more difficult will be identification of the Central Nervous System (CNS), the Autonomic Nervous System (ANS) and related mechanical and neuroendocrine processes operating during interactive effects as well as gaining a precise understanding of how such processes are related to pathophysiological mechanisms in atherogenesis and clinical CHD. At the very least, new findings in this arena offer more evidence of the importance of primary and secondary prevention programs. In designing such programs, one might well consider that the two separate categories of risk factors (physical and psychosocial) are not so separate after all. (p. 19)

The postulation of a proper model for the interaction of risk factors is vital for the appreciation of statistical calculations such as those quoted from the U.S. Surgeon General, or the Royal College of Physicians. In the absence of such a model, the figures are meaningless, even if cause of death had been reliably assessed (which it had not) and even if a proper method of calculating causal determination from statistical association had been established (which it had not). On all these grounds, then, one must conclude that the figures for deaths from smoking, so often publicized, have no scientific basis. It is unfortunate that official publications usually just repeat the kinds of calculations discussed here and fail to answer legitimate criticisms or to spell out the precise nature of the models of interaction assumed. It is difficult to understand this reluctance to accept the existence of problems and anomalies in the argument that smoking causes disease or to deal constructively with objections. The issue is of fundamental importance socially, medically, and scientifically and should be so treated.

These inadmissible projections derived from faulty data have been taken up with enthusiasm by the media, which, taking these estimates seriously, have sensationalized these improbable and unproven estimates to an extent that has convinced large numbers of lay people, and also medical professionals not intimately familiar with the evidence, that, indeed, smoking is responsible for a large majority of the deaths from cancer and CHD. Clark (1989) has demonstrated very clearly, by an analysis of the way the topic has been treated by quality papers, that the journalists involved abandoned objectivity and that a bandwaggon effect was created, which in turn promoted medical efforts to find more and better evidence for these doubtful propositions. As Clark points out, there was an almost complete absence of reports of a controversy in this field and a complete avoidance of balance concerning such issues as public smoking, passive smoking, and tobacco sponsorship in advertising.

This lack of objectivity is a serious matter in issues concerning general health questions, but it may have more serious implications, as indicated in an article by Grossarth-Maticek and Eysenck (1989a), suggesting that media information that smoking causes illness can become a self-fulfilling prophecy. The study found that smokers who obtained their information concerning the possible deleterious effects of smoking on health from the media only showed a significantly higher death rate than did smokers who derived this information from self-observation or who did not believe it. Thus, the extremely one-sided way in which the media have treated this issue shows a lack of responsibility, which may itself cause stress and through stress, increase the chances of people who derive their information from the media to die of cancer and CHD.

In this introductory chapter, I have not attempted to discuss evidence suggesting that writers supporting to orthodox view are not entirely along the right lines or to refute evidence concerning the claims that smoking causes deaths from cancer and CHD or that passive smoking has similar effects (Saracci & Riboli, 1989); this is accomplished in later chapters. In this section, I intend merely to draw attention to the fact that there is an ongoing debate concerning different models of interaction between risk factors and disease and that the existence of such a debate has been almost completely disregarded by the media and even by authoritative publications by the Royal College of Medicine in the United Kingdom, the Surgeon General in the United States, and the World Health Organization. As mentioned, the estimates of the number of lives that could be saved if only people would quit smoking or never take it up have little scientific basis, and again, this will be documented in later chapters.

The next chapter concerns the question of the empirical evidence about the effects of giving up smoking and the extent to which this evidence supports the "orthodox" view. The validity of the evidence concerning a statistical relationship between smoking and disease will then be examined in more detail, and the acceptability of a causal inference concerning this relationship will be discussed.

2
Does Quitting Smoking Save Lives?

Claims like those of the U.S. Surgeon General (1982) that giving up smoking lowers lung cancer and other types of mortality are, of course, vital for any consideration of possible relations between smoking, cancer, and coronary heart disease (CHD). There are two ways of studying such effects. The first takes a sample of subjects, usually relatively homogeneous (e.g., British physicians), follows them up, and examines the death rates from various causes of those who give up smoking and those who continue to smoke (Doll & Peto, 1976). The alternative method is to form two groups, matched on as many relevant variables as possible, and to consider one of these as a control, receiving no instruction, while the other is a therapy group receiving instruction to give up smoking and possibly also receiving advice relating to other risk factors, such as poor diet, high blood pressure, and so on. Unfortunately, practically all the positive results of giving up smoking have been reported from studies using the first of these methods, that is, self-selection, and it is widely recognized that no relevant conclusions regarding causality can be drawn from studies of self-selected populations only. It is now quite clear that this is a crucial factor, making it impossible to compare ex-smokers and continuing smokers with the aim of establishing the causal link between smoking and disease.

G.D. Friedman, Siegelaub, Dales, and Seltzer (1979) have shown that ex-smokers and continuing smokers are already very different from the point of view of health at the time that the ex-smokers give up smoking, and Eysenck (1980) has shown that with respect to personality, ex-smokers are more like nonsmokers than they are like continuing smokers. Thus, the necessary conditions for the paradigm are not fulfilled, namely, that ex-smokers and continuing smokers should be similar or identical from the point of view of personality and health at the time that ex-smokers give up smoking. It follows that *no* interpretation along causal lines can be made of the differential mortality rate of ex-smokers and continuing smokers.

Quitters are Different from Continuing Smokers

The Friedman et al. (1979) study is particularly important in demonstrating the lack of comparability between smokers who continue to smoke and smokers who quit smoking. The study concerns white and black men and women who had had three or more examinations concerning their health. The authors compared ex-smokers and continuing smokers for a large number of characteristics associated with risk of CHD; assessments of these characteristics were made at a time when all were smoking cigarettes. Persons who remained non-smokers provided an additional comparison group. The authors found that smokers who later quit showed statistically significant differences from smokers who continued smoking in certain cardiovascular symptoms, social and personal characteristics, smoking intensity, and some other traits. Compared with persistent smokers, quitters in most or all race–sex subgroups had higher relative weight and lower alcohol consumption but smoked fewer cigarettes for shorter duration; inhaled less; had higher vital capacity; lower leukocyte count; lower prevalence of abnormal electrocardiogram findings; less exertional chest pain, exertional dyspnea, and exertional leg pain; high educational level; and a tendency to answer a psychological questionnaire less like persons who later developed myocardial infarction. Other CHD-related characteristics such as cholesterol and blood pressure showed small differences. It is important to note that controlling for smoking quantity had little effect on differences between the persistent quitters and persistent smokers for certain characteristics that seemed likely to be smoking related. For several characteristics, quitters were more similar at index examination to never smokers than to persistent smokers. Similar results were obtained in the famous Framingham study, although the numbers involved were too small to give incontrovertible evidence. In all instances, persistent smokers and quitters had directional differences similar to those found in the Friedman et al. study.

The results of this study (Friedman et al. 1979) should not be taken to mean that follow-up studies of self-selected quitters and smokers do not give important information. The study merely suggests that the situation is a very complex one and that detailed medical and psychological examinations must be made of quitters and consistent smokers *before* the former quit smoking. A complex statistical inquiry could then be undertaken to estimate the degree to which quitting had an effect independent of the already existing differences in disease-related characteristics. Methodologically, existing studies leaving out this consideration must be somewhat flawed. It is unfortunate that many publications draw conclusions from these studies without mentioning the contamination pointed out by Friedman et al. or the necessity of taking these considerations into account.

The MRFIT Study

From a general point of view, the study of the Multiple Risk Factor Intervention Trial (MRFIT) Research Group (1982) is an example of the type of study of groups that are not self-selected but include a measure of randomization. In this randomized primary prevention trial to test the effect of a multifactor intervention program on mortality from CHD, 12,866 high-risk men aged 35 to 57 years were randomly assigned either to a special intervention program consisting of drug-care treatment for hypertension, counseling for cigarette smoking, and dietary advice for lowering blood cholesterol levels, *or* to the usual resources of health care in the community. An average follow-up period of 7 years showed that risk-factor levels declined in both group but to a significantly greater degree for the experimental group. Mortality from CHD was 17.9/1,000 in the experimental group and 19.3/1,000 in the control group, a statistically nonsignificant difference. Total mortality rates were 41.2/1,000 in the experimental group and 40.4/1,000 in the control group; that is, mortality was greater in the experimental than in the control group. Thus, the effect of significantly lowering the consumption of cigarettes (as well as significantly lowering blood cholesterol levels and also lowering blood pressure) was practically nonexistent; the slightly greater mortality rate for the experimental group was not statistically significant. The results concerning CHD are discussed again later; the overall mortality rate, however, is important because it includes cancers and should have declined as a consequence of the lower levels of cigarette consumption in the experimental group. This is important in view of the statement made in the U.S. Surgeon General's Report (1982) that "cigarette smokers have overall mortality rates substantially greater than those of non-smokers" (p. 5) and that it would be expected that giving up cigarette smoking would reduce these overall mortality rates. Apparently, this is not so overall, and, as other studies have shown, it is not so with respect to cancers specifically.

Attempts (e.g., Oliver, 1982) to explain away the disappointing results of course have been made, and the $115 million experiment is certainly subject to criticism. Jarvis, West, Tunstall-Pedoe, & Vesey, 1984 have criticized, particularly, the methods used to measure smoking activity. Moreover, the study lacked appropriate psychological expertise in looking at stress and personality factors that are known to influence the outcome (Eysenck, 1985). Nevertheless, the study does show that even on such a very large scale, there is no evidence of any effects for cessation of smoking to increase chances of survival. The data have been analyzed for small subgroups, with slightly more positive outcome, but such a procedure is statistically inadmissible when the overall result does not significantly bear out the theories under investigation, or even shows opposite outcome.

The latest follow-up of the MRFIT study gives results after 10.5 years (Multiple Risk Factor Intervention Trial Research Group, 1990). The results were somewhat better when comparing the special intervention (SI) with the usual sources of health care (UC) group; however, "the more favourable mortality experience for SI compared with UC men after 1982 was observed primarily for men with hypertension at baseline" (p. 1799), that is, among men at special risk. There are many oddities in the results. Thus, there were "slightly more deaths in the SI group than the UC group due to other ischaemic heart disease (96 vs. 86 deaths)" (p. 1799), a phenomenon also observed in the Hypertension Detection and Follow-up Program (1988). Similarly, neoplastic disease of the respiratory and intrathoracic organs showed 66 deaths in the SI group but only 55 in the UC group. Again, "Results for men with resting ECG abnormalities at baseline are in marked contrast to those for men without such abnormalities. . . . Reasons for the higher SI than UC mortality in this sub-group remain unclear." (p. 1799.) All neoplastic deaths show hardly any difference between SI and UC: 140 deaths compared with 149 deaths, respectively, a negligible difference. There is thus much confusion in this latest report, which possibly is due in part to the failure of the analyses to take into account synergistic effects of multiple risk factors discussed elsewhere in this book. For initially healthy people, that is, not suffering from hypertension, there is little effect overall.

The data may go some way to indicate that lowering blood pressure does reduce the risk of heart attack, in spite of the large number of negative results in the past (Collins et al., 1990; MacMahon et al., 1990). These meta-analyses attempt to show positive results by aggregating all published data, in spite of important methodological and other differences; such a procedure is of course improper and unlikely to give useful results (Eysenck, 1984).

MRFIT Is Not Alone!

It should be noted that other trials, such as the continuing World Health Organization European Trial, which comprises 63,733 men aged 49 to 59 in 44 factories in Britain, Belgium, Italy, Poland, and Spain (World Health Organization European Collaborative Group, 1982) also make depressing reading in that changes were smaller than expected and not completely consistent or sustained. The authors found that, despite an estimated fall of 14% in CHD risk in the whole group and of 24% in the high-risk subgroup after 4 years, no equivalent fall in the incidence of CHD was shown even in a study of this size. Similarly, in the North Karelia project (Puska, Tuamilehito, & Saloney, 1979), an overall mean net reduction of 17% in men and of 12% in women occurred 5 years after inception with regard to quitting cigarette smoking, reducing blood pressure, and plasma cholesterol concentrations in the intervention community, compared with the control community; but here also there was no reduction in mortality from CHD. Only the small-scale Oslo study (Holme, 1982) succeeded in showing a reduction in the incidence of CHD with cessation of smoking and dietary intervention to lower lipid concentrations in non-hypertensive men in high-risk categories. This combination of smoking cessation and cholesterol reduction makes interpretation difficult. Overall, the outlook is not promising, although better-designed, better-controlled, and longer-continued studies might alter the outlook. All one can say is that attempts to prove the influence of cigarette smoking as a causal factor in disease by means of trials avoiding the obvious error of self-selection have not on the whole been successful.

In addition to the trials mentioned, in several others, such as the Oslo study (Leren et al., 1975) and the Finnish Businessmen's study (Miettinen et al., 1985), smoking reduced groups were compared with control groups. In the six major studies, none showed a significant difference in total mortality, CHD mortality, or cancer mortality. So much for the alleged beneficial effects on mortality of giving up smoking!

Methodologically superior to any of these studies is a report by Rose and Hamilton (1978), in which a randomized controlled trial of smoking cessation is reported for 1,445 male smokers aged 40 to 59 at high risk of cardiorespiratory disease. Marked differences in amount of smoking were observed in the intervention groups, as compared with the control group; 51% of the intervention group reported that they were not smoking any cigarettes, and most of the others reported a reduction. Nevertheless, as the authors report, "Disappointingly, we find no evidence at all of any reduction in total mortality" (p. 280). They did find some improvements in minor symptoms, such as coughing, and in chronic sputum production in men with early chronic bronchitis; many also reported a lessening of dyspnea, but airways obstruction did not improve.

The studies mentioned have all dealt mainly with CHD, and it might be thought that the results might not apply to lung cancer. However, Rose, Hamilton, Colvell, and Shipley (1982) report a 10-year follow-up study of middle-aged male smokers at high risk of cardiorespiratory disease who were allocated randomly to an intervention or a normal-care group. The intensive advice given to the first group was successful in reducing the average consumption of cigarettes by just over one half in this group. For the normal care group of 731 men, the authors reported 25 cases of lung cancer; in the intervention group of 714, they reported 22 comparable cases—a nonsignificant difference. Data for all deaths in these groups are free from diagnostic error and are hence the most reliable: 17.2% in the intervention group died compared with 17.5% in the normal-care group, giving a negligible and statistically nonsignificant difference. Thus, this study gives results similar to the other intervention studies using randomized groups—a failure to detect any effect of giving up smoking.

Curiously, Rose et al. found at a significant level ($p < .003$) of higher rates among the intervention group subjects of "all cancers other than lung cancer" compared with the nonintervention group subjects; whether this result can be replicated is, of course, another matter, particularly because there are difficulties in assigning a valid probability value to an a posteriori hypothesis. Burch (1983) comments that, for all these studies, the results for total mortality are entirely in line with the analysis of temporal trends of sex- and age-specific mortality from all causes in England and Wales, which "failed to detect any causal influence of cigarette smoking when consumption was rising and no prophylactic influence when consumption was falling" (p. 832).

A relevant study was carried out by Grossarth-Maticek and Eysenck (unpublished) as part of a series of prospective studies described in detail in Chapter 7. Out of a much larger group, we selected 138 continuing male smokers and 138 matched male quitters. The matching was by age (55.3 or 55.4 years) and stress–personality, using a typology explicated in Chapter 6. Based on that typology, half of the sample were cancer prone, half CHD prone. All had smoked between 20 and 30 cigarettes per day for ove 20 years, and the quitters had given up completely between 10 and 15 years at the time of the study. Thirteen years later, mortality was established for members for both groups, with the results shown in Table 1.

Table 1 shows no suggestive differences between the two groups concerning total mortality or any particular mortality. If anything, smokers have slightly lower mortality than quitters, but of course, the difference is statistically quite insignificant. This study thus confirms results from several other studies emphasizing the lack of effect on mortality of giving up smoking. It is difficult to accomodate these data in any of the current models, but it seems possible that the biological effects of smoking may follow a negatively accelerated growth curve nearing its asymptote after 1 or 2 years, with smoking thereafter or quitting making no difference. These biological effects then combine with other risk factors (stress, personality, genetic predisposition) to produce medical effects. This model has the

TABLE 1. Mortality cause and rate among smokers and quitters at 13-year follow-up

Cause of death	Smokers	Quitters
Coronary heart disease	16	14
Lung cancer	8	5
Other cancers	19	25
Other causes	17	18
Still living	78	76
Total	138	138

great virtue of also accounting for the lack of a dose–response relation between number of years smoked and probability of disease; this curious lack is discussed in Chaper 4. It also accounts for the observed dose–response relationship between number of cigarettes smoked per day and disease if one assumes that the asymptote of the growth curve is determined by the number of cigarettes smoked per day. Some such model as this is the only one to account for several apparently contradictory facts; it deserves direct empirical study to show whether it can be confirmed or disproved. (Some evidence for the model is found in Chapters 6 and 7).

I have not reviewed all the many studies looking at the effects of cessation of smoking on CHD, but such a summary has recently been published by McCormick and Skrabanek (1988), under the challenging title "Coronary Heart Disease Is Not Preventable by Population Interventions." As they point out, "This review of the present experimental evidence that we can prevent much coronary heart disease provides no data to justify the time, energy, and money which are being devoted to this crusade. . . . to base population strategies on unproven hypotheses seems unreasonable" (p. 841). Several authors (e.g., Fries, Green, & Lavine, 1985; Gunning-Schepers, Barrendregt, & Maas, 1989) have tried to point out certain redeeming features in the evidence, but they do not seriously deny the major conclusion in the McCormick and Skrabanek study.

It is interesting to note that well-meant suggestions based on ignorance or faulty research studies may in fact decrease rather than increase survival. Thus, consider the recommendation that one should seriously lower one's cholesterol level through diet changes or drugs, in order to reduce the incidence of CHD. Yet cholesterol plays a vital role within the body, and reductions in cholesterol level may have disastrous consequences. Oliver (1988) has recently reviewed the literature and concludes that "reducing cholesterol does not reduce mortality" (p. 814). He finds that the evidence shows an *inverse* relation between serum cholesterol and cancer, which might or might not be causal. He shows that "the frequent claims that thousands of lives will be saved by reducing plasma cholesterol are unsubstantiated" and explains that "most extrapolations from epidemiologic data and simulation models fail to take into account the differential effect that cholesterol reduction seems to have on each of the three main end points—non-fatal cardiac events, cardiac deaths and non-cardiovascular deaths" (p. 815). Finally, he warns against the evangelical publicity campaigns that are being waged in favor of cholesterol reduction; as he says, "The issue is a very serious one if vast sums are spent and widespread changes are made in the lifestyle of normal people when the accumulated evidence is that total mortality is unchanged or possibly even increased" (p. 815). *Mutatis mutandis*, much the same could be said about the antismoking campaigns!

The position is starkly clarified in a meta-analysis of all large primary prevention trials involving randomized clinical intervention aimed at the reduction of cholesterol, either by diet change, drug administration, or both, including a control group, and successful in achieving such reduction as compared with the control group (Muldoon, Manuck, & Matthews, 1990). Altogether, 24,847 men participated, with follow-up periods totaling 119,000 person-years, during which 1,147 deaths occurred. None of the studies, singly or in combination, provided evidence of lowered mortality in the intervention group. A slight reduction in CHD mortality was almost exactly counter balanced by an increase in deaths from suicide or violence, apparent in all studies and hence not a statistical accident. As Muldoon et al. state, several clinical studies have reported low serum cholesterol concentrations among criminals, people with diagnoses of violent or aggressive conduct disorders, homicidal offenders with histories of violence and suicide attempts related to alcohol, and people with poorly internalized social norms and low self-control. Cancer mortality was also raised in the intervention group, but it seems likely that this was due to the carcinogenic action of some of the drugs prescribed.

An important point here clearly relates to the relationship, emphasized throughout this book, between physical and psychosocial factors in mortality. The relationship between low cholesterol and high aggressiveness and violence is as important socially as the relationship between high cholesterol and CHD.

Smoking Effects in Different Populations

One further point relating to non-smoking as a defense against disease may be mentioned, namely, the suggestion that there is a correspondence of lung cancer mortality among different populations with different tobacco consumption rates (Lyon, Gardner, & West, 1980). The point Lyon et al. made is that Mormons and Californian Seventh Day Adventists, non-smoking groups, have low incidence of lung cancer.

The membership of such groups, of course, involves self-selection, or descent from self-selected progenitors, but even overlooking this obvious point, the results present difficulties for the orthodox view, as Enstrom (1980) concluded after a careful examination of the evidence. According to the simple causal hypothesis, Mormons, who refrain from smoking in accordance with the dictates of their religion, should have an incidence of lung cancer the same as that found in comparable nonsmokers of the general population. Lyon et al. (1980) compared the incidence in Mormons with that in non-Mormons (smokers and nonsmokers) in Utah over the period 1967 to 1975, finding an age-adjusted incidence of lung cancer in male Mormons of 46% of that in male non-Mormons; for females the incidence was 44%. Comparing the Mormons with non-smokers only, it appears that, on the basis of the orthodox view, the incidence of lung cancer in male Mormons is at least twice that expected for a population of nonsmokers who are not Mormons. "On the constitutional hypothesis, the Mormon population—involving selection—comprises a mixture of never-smoking and smoking genotypes with, among males at least, a relatively high proportion of the former" (Burch, 1983, p. 832). The cancer mortality patterns in Mormons are "not clearly explained by their smoking habits" (Enstrom, 1980).

Actually, a suitable use of published data comparing Utah matched with other states can be used to test the hypothesis that a 50% lower rate of smoking and drinking would save large numbers of lives. The following calculations are quoted from an unpublished analysis by Dr. Miron Johnston (personal communication, January 1988):

The low mortality rate in Utah (5.5 deaths per 1000 population, as compared with 8.7 for the total U.S.) is often cited as "proof" that abstention from alcohol, tobacco and caffeine puts the Mormons in Utah at considerably lower than average risk of premature death. (Per capita beer and cigarette consumption in Utah is consistently about half that of the total U.S.).

Low *crude* mortality rates must be corrected for age differences and racial composition. Using age-specific mortality rates and comparing Utah with the Plain States (North and South Dakota, Nebraska, Kansas, Minnesota, and Iowa), which resemble Utah demographically in terms of climate, ethnic mix, and population density, one can obtain figures freed of these obvious contaminating factors. These figures still contain deaths that are due to alcohol abuse (i.e., deaths due to drunk driving, alcohol-caused liver disease, etc.). This leaves only 4,173 premature deaths among white men attributable to a combination of caffeine, tobacco, and alcohol used in moderation. (From this one should probably subtract at least some of the 9,826 deaths among white men under age 75 attributed to cirrhosis of the liver and other unspecified chronic liver diseases without mention of alcohol, a frequent omission on death certificates!) Such a difference, less than 4,173 deaths, is minute, considering the very large numbers involved, even if one disregards the final correction suggested; it gives no support to the suggestion of hundreds of thousands whose lives could be saved by abstinence from smoking! Thus, a realistic comparison of populations differing in smoking and drinking habits by some 50% suggests a negligible difference in mortality.

Just as the alleged effects of smoking have ended in disarray, so have the alleged effects of diet on CHD. Already in the late 1970s, Mann (1977) and J. McMichael (1979) announced "an end of an era" and held an inquest "on the topic." As the latter points out, "all well-controlled trials of cholesterol reducing diets and drugs have failed to reduce coronary (CHD) mortality and morbidity" (p. 173). More recent studies, using new and more effective drugs, might lead to a less pessimistic view. Recognition is now dawning that a low-fat diet, concentrated in polyunsaturated fats, may even be harmful in inducing cancer, although the evidence for this does not at present seem strong enough to formulate any conclusions (Schatzkin et al., 1988). Le Fanu (1987) has pointed out that medical advice based on so-called epidemiological evidence follows fads that are often contradictory, not based on proper scientific evidence, finally fail, and are succeeded by other fads. The possibility cannot be ruled out that the antismoking campaign may be such another fad. Certainly, there is no evidence in the studies reviewed that quitting smoking has any strong beneficial effects on survival or on the avoidance of cancer and CHD. As Burch (1986) has put the question: "Can epidemiology become a rigorous science?" (p. 956). On the basis of the existing evidence, one would hesitate to give a positive answer to the question.

One further study deserves special mention here because of the rather paradoxical results and also because of the well-deserved fame this study has received as a function of its methodological excellence. The study is the Framingham Heart Study. In 1974, Gordon, Kannel, and McGee (1974) reported data for a 12-year follow-up study. For male cigarette smokers, aged 45 to 74 at entry, who subsequently stopped smoking, the incidence rate for CHD (other than angina pectoris) was found to be "half that experienced by those who continued to smoke." This finding has become the most widely quoted evidence for the belief that stopping smoking dramatically reduces the risk of CHD.

As Seltzer (1989) has pointed out, however, this evidence (Gordon et al., 1974) is seriously compromised by an important omission. In the comparison of risk for continuing and quitting smokers, no data were cited

TABLE 2. Comparison of coronary heart disease (CHD) morbidity ratios and incidence rates of never smokers and ex-smokers at various years of follow-up

Follow-up (years)	Morbidity ratios[a] or incidence rate		Proportionate difference
9.1	Never smokers	77	+67%
	Past smokers	46	
12 ("heart attacks")	Never smokers	82	+39%
	Ex-smokers	59	
16	Never smokers	91	+49%
	Ex-smokers	61	
18 ("heart attacks")	Never smokers	17.7[b]	+36%
	Ex-smokers	13.0[b]	
22	Never smokers	29.8[b]	+23%
	Ex-smokers	24.2[b]	

Note. Data from "Framingham Study Data and 'Established Wisdom' About Cigarette Smoking and Coronary Heart Disease" by C.C. Seltzer, 1989, Journal of Clinical Epidemiology, 42, p. 747.
Copyright 1989 by Pergamon Press PLC.
Reprinted by permission of the publisher and author.
[a] Ratio of observed to expected rate (100 times those observed divided by those expected).
[b] CHD incidence rates per 100 men.

for the analogous heart attack rate of never smokers. Seltzer obtained evidence on this point for various follow-up periods, and the results are shown in Table 2. It can be seen that the CHD rate was higher for never smokers than for ex-smokers; at a 12-year follow-up point, the age-adjusted incidence of CHD was 8.3/100 for ex-smokers and 12.0/100 for never smokers. Four additional analyses at various follow-up points are given in Table 2, showing that the CHD rates for never smokers are from 23% to 67% proportionately higher than for ex-smokers. These results are truly extraordinary and completely contradict the view that smoking causes CHD and that giving up smoking will improve one's chances of survival. Such a hypothesis requires a linear relationship between never smoking, quitting, and continuing to smoke; the existence of a very strong curvilinear relationship makes any such interpretation impossible.

3
How Strong is the Association Between Smoking and Disease?

So far I have taken for granted the existence of a strong statistical relationship between cigarette smoking and disease, particularly cancer and CHD. Such a relationship can be demonstrated along two rather different lines. The first of these is the cross-sectional method. Here one studies a group of patients suffering from a given disease and compares them with some form of control group that may be suffering from a different type of disease, or no disease at all, with respect to smoking habits. This method is obviously weak methodologically. The choice of a control group is clearly crucial, but any particular choice may be faulted for a variety of reasons. The method depends a good deal on memory (When did you take up smoking? How many cigarettes did you smoke? What types of cigarettes did you smoke?), and memory is known to be faulty and subject to falsification. The method has many other weaknesses, which are discussed later. Few epidemiologists would doubt that the second method to be discussed, namely, the prospective study, is superior because it is not subject to these weaknesses.

The Framingham Heart Study

In a prospective study, a sample is chosen at a point in time, A, and followed up over varying periods of time; at time B, the examiner inquires into the health status of the probands and ascertains deaths and cause of death, or incidence, as the case might be. This method also has weaknesses (probands may be lost through emigration, or they may refuse to allow doctors to discuss incidence, etc.), but these can usually be controlled statistically or avoided in one way or another.

The most important follow-up study to have been undertaken is undoubtedly the Framingham Heart Study, which has been called the "cornerstone" of coronary heart disease (CHD) epidemiology (Leaventon 1987). This study covers more than three decades of surveillance of a substantial cohort of men and women and has produced a mountain of data and several hundred publications. The leading Framington Study investigators have interpreted the follow-up data on the relationship between smoking and CHD in a very positive manner, declaring that cigarette smoking is a "powerful contributor" to the cause of CHD (Dawber, 1980; Kannel, 1981). The refrain has been taken up by almost all commentators, and the Framingham Study is universally regarded as the strongest proof of the existence of an important and significant relationship between smoking and CHD.

The study cohort was obtained from a random subsample of the adult residents of Framingham, Massachusetts; the response rate was 69%. There was in addition a group of volunteers, whose differences from the originally sampled group were not considered to be important (Dawber, 1980). The final cohort consisted of 2,282 men and 2,845 women, who were aged 29 through 62 years and free from CHD at the initial examination. Members of the study received a standarized cardiovascular examination at entry, including information on habits, physical characteristics, and blood chemistry. Data so acquired included information on tobacco smoking, alcohol consumption, systolic and diastolic blood pressure, hematocrit, hemoglobin, serum cholesterol, phospholipids, uric acid, relative weight, vital capacity, electrocardiogram, and urinalysis for sugar and albumin.

After the initiation, participants were checked for cardiovascular disease every 2 years, in an investigation that included medical history, physical examination, blood and other laboratory tests, with CHD episodes classified as myocardial infarction, angina pectoris, coronary insufficiency, sudden death, or CHD deaths. The follow-up period now extends over 30 years, and a large number of data are available to answer the question of the relationship between cigarette smoking and CHD. Seltzer (1989) has conducted such an examination of the existing data.

Table 3 shows the major results of Seltzer's (1989) investigation. The important columns are those showing risk ratios, that is, the ratio of cigarette smokers to nonsmokers in the incidence of CHD. The ratio of 1.0 indicates no relationship whatsoever between smoking and CHD; a risk ratio below 1.0 indicates that smoking actually benefitted probands, whereas risk ratios above 1.0 indicate that smoking was somehow linked with CHD. The risk ratio of 2 has been designated by Hutchinson (1968) and Wynder (1987) as the boundary of a weak association.

Table 3 shows that for women, there is either no relationship at all between smoking and CHD or an inverse one; several of the risk ratio variables are below 1.0. Clearly, there is no evidence here for any relationship between smoking and CHD. For the men, the values are slightly above 1.0, although for the 30-year follow-up, using the total set of age groups from 35 to 84 years, the ratio is exactly 1.0, suggesting that if there is any relationship, it is very weak indeed, falling well below the 2.0 level. Thus, the best and most frequently cited evidence for the notion that cigarette smoking is a powerful contributor to the cause of CHD completely fails

TABLE 3. Coronary heart disease (CHD) risk ratios (cigarette smokers compared with nonsmokers) calculated from the Framingham Heart Study incidence data

Follow-up (years)	Incidence	Ages	Nonsmoker classification for comparison with smokers[b]	Risk Ratios Men	Risk Ratios Women
9.1	After exam 1	40–59	Never smokers	1.5[c]	—
			Nonsmokers (never, past, less than half per day)	1.8[c]	—
12	After exam 1	30–59	Noncigarette	1.8[d]	1.0[d]
14	After exam 1	35–64	None	1.4	.9
16	After exam 1	35–64	None	1.3	.9
	Average annual incidence rate	35–74	None	1.3	.8
18	Average annual incidence rate	45–74	None	1.3	1.0
20	Average annual "smoothed" rate	45–74	None	1.4	—
22	After exam 1	30–59	Noncigarette	1.3	.8
24	After exam 1	30–59	Noncigarette	1.3	.9
26	After exam 1	35–84	Noncigarette	1.3[e]	—
30	Average annual incidence rate	35–64	None	1.6	1.1
		35–74		1.3	1.0
		35–84		1.0	1.0

Note. Data from "Framingham Study Data and 'Established Wisdom' About Cigarette Smoking and Coronary Heart Disease" by C.C. Seltzer, 1989, Journal of Clinical Epidemiology, 42, p. 747.
Copyright 1989 by Pergamon Press PLC.
Reprinted by permission of the publisher and author.
[a] Age-adjusted by assigning equal weights to rates in each age groups, in accordance with the Framingham method listed in Table 2.
[b] Framingham categories of "none" and "noncigarette" include ex-smokers, and pipe and cigar smokers in addition to "never smokers."
[c] "Standardized incidence ratios" with CHD limited to nonfatal and fatal myocardial infarction and sudden CHD death.
[d] Framingham "morbidity ratios."
[e] Framingham "coronary morbidity."

to live up to this description; it shows that at best there is a very weak relationship for men and none whatsoever for women.

Would the relationship be stronger for heavy smokers? It is possible that the relationship there might have been obscured by large numbers of light smokers, but this does not seem to be so. Smokers of 40 or more cigarettes per day were found to have a CHD risk ratio of only 1.3 (Kannel & Gordon, 1970).

When associations are weak, it is an elementary rule that one should look for possible confounding factors. A search for such confounding factors would have to take into account the fact that Hopkins and Williams (1981) listed 246 suggested coronary risk factors in their survey! Only a few of these, of course, are available on the Framingham protocols. Seltzer (1989) carried out a multivariable analysis including, as previous analyses had not, data about type A personality, which is believed to be CHD prone, and when such psychosocial factors were included along with systolic blood pressure and serum cholesterol, *cigarette smoking was not found to be a significant predictor of CHD or myocardial infarction in men or of CHD or angina pectoris in women.* (Psychosocial factors and type A personality are discussed in Chapter 6.) The Framingham investigators also found that cigarette smoking does not make an independent contribution to cardiovascular disease when fibrinogen is considered along with standard Framingham risk factors (Kannel, O'Agostino, & Belanger, 1987). Seltzer (1989) makes an interesting comparison of the conclusions of the U.S. Surgeon General's reports on "cardiovascular disease" (1983) and the conclusions to be drawn from the Framingham Study. The major conclusion of the 1983 report is that "cigarette smoking is a major cause of coronary heart disease in the U.S. for both men and women." This conclusion is supported by the following statements:

1. In men, the incidence of CHD is two fold greater in cigarette smokers than in nonsmokers and fourfold greater in heavy smokers.
2. In women, the rates of CHD are lower than in men but are commensurately higher when the smoking patterns are similar to those in men.
3. The risk of developing CHD increases with the duration (in years) of cigarette smoking.
4. The cessation of smoking leads to CHD death rates that are substantially lower in the stopped smokers than are in the continuing

TABLE 4. Comparison of U.S. Surgeon General's coronary heart disease (CHD) findings and those of the Framingham Study data with respect to cigarette smoking

Criteria	U.S. Surgeon General's findings	Framingham data findings
Men		
Univariate association	Strong	Weak
Multivariate association	Strong	Non-significant; absent
Women		
Univariate association	Present, but less than in men	Absent
Multivariate association	Present	Absent
Duration of cigarette smoking	Increase of CHD with increase of duration of smoking	Absent
Cessation of cigarette smoking	Gradual reduction of CHD to level of nonsmokers	Immediate reduction of CHD to level below that of never smokers

Note. Data from "Framingham Stidy Data and 'Established Wisdom' About Cigarette Smoking and Coronary Heart Disease" by C.C. Seltzer, 1989, *Journal of Clinical Epidemiology, 42,* p. 747.
Copyright 1989 by Pergamon Press PLC.
Adapted by permission.

smokers, and after 10 years of nonsmoking, the CHD incidence of former light smokers approximates those of nonsmokers.

Seltzer (1989) developed a table (Table 4) that makes interesting reading. As Seltzer points out:

The Surgeon-General's views and other features of the "conventional wisdom" about cigarette smoking and coronary heart disease obviously depend on many other studies beyond those of the Framingham cohort, and on many other data that have not been cited here for the smoking/coronary heart disease relationship. The main purpose of this paper is simply to point out that for the critical relationships noted here, the Framingham data substantially disagree with the "conventional wisdom" and that the anomaly remains unexplained. Because of the unusual care and thoroughness with which the Framingham cohort was selected, followed, and examined, it is difficult to attribute the anomaly to some intrinsic error in Framingham's epidemiologic methods. The explanation for the discrepancy is an intriguing challenge for future research.

Statistics and Statistics

The finding in the Framingham Study that there is a very weak association, if any, between smoking and CHD makes it desirable to look at the possible strength of a relationship between smoking and smoking-associated diseases in the form of a meta-analysis, that is, averaging across all available materials. Wakefield (1988) collected and reviewed empirical studies from the 1985 *Smoking and Health Abstracts*. The quality of the methods employed in each study was rated by two doctors of experimental psychology who did not know the authors or the results of the studies they rated. The relationships between smoking and the health variable (S) in each study were converted to a standard effect size and correlated for comparison. Results were presented for 10 categories of health variables. The relationships between smoking and health were small for all categories, with an overall relationship equivalent to a correlation of 0.13. Poorer studiers yielded larger relationships between smoking and health than did methodologically stronger studies. A similar analysis of the 1982 Surgeon General's report produced an overall correlation of 0.17 between smoking and cancer. The relationship between smoking and disease as shown in recent empirical investigations is very weak and would be even weaker if only methodologically adequate studies were considered.

As Wakefield (1988) points out, a major problem with the literature is its consistent reliance on the concept of the relative risk of a disease for smokers and nonsmokers. Relative risk is conceptually the quotient of the probability of a disease for smokers and the probability of the disease for nonsmokers, and is interpreted as the number of times the risk for nonsmokers is increased for smokers (Fleiss, 1987). Usually computed by the "odds ratio," relative risk is a concept that is useful primarily for educational purposes rather than as a measure of the degree of association between two variables (i.e., smoking and disease). Relative risk allows an understandable way of communicating the "odds" involved in relationships between variables to persons with little or no statistical background; however, for conditions with small probabilities of occurrence, as is the case with most diseases, relative risk may be large, and consequently frightening, numbers resulting from trivial relationships. For example, five times a very small probability of developing a disease is still a very small probability of developing the disease. A better way of measuring the degree of relationship between two variables is with a correlation coefficient that expresses "no relationship" as a 0, and a "perfect relationship" as a 1.

The near zero effects for smoking and health variables estimated from all available literature abstracted in 1985 suggest an explanation of health problems in terms of simple causation by smoking is no longer plausible. Other alternatives, including personality, stress, genetic factors, and general lifestyle as leading to health problems. . . . must now be considered more plausible than smoking. (Wakefield, 1988, p. 473).

It is impossible in the limited space here to discuss all the many studies in this field. More detailed discussions are available (Eysenck, 1980, 1986). Instead, following is a more general discussion of the available methodologies and the type of error that is so characteristic of much of the work undertaken in trying to discover the relationship between smoking and disease.

Overall correlations of a size between .13 and .17, as discovered in the Wakefield (1988) analysis, are much too weak to be taken very seriously, particularly because univariate studies of this kind cannot in the nature of things take into account other factors that may influence both the variables correlated. As Seltzer (1989) has shown in connection with the Framingham Study, when even a small number of other variables are taken into account, the apparent correlation between smoking and disease vanishes completely. The obvious fact that there are many risk factors in cancer and CHD makes univariate analysis pointless, yet the vast majority of studies have failed to employ the required multivariate paradigm.

Multivariate Paradigm

One of the reasons why a multivariate paradigm is so necessary concerns the nomological network of intercorrelated factors that appears in every large-scale investigation of risk factors associated with smoking. Thus, smoking is connected with personality, as discussed in Chapter 6, and it is also correlated with drinking, antisocial behavior, low IQ, sexual behavior, and many other variables (Eysenck, 1980). Figure 1, to take but one

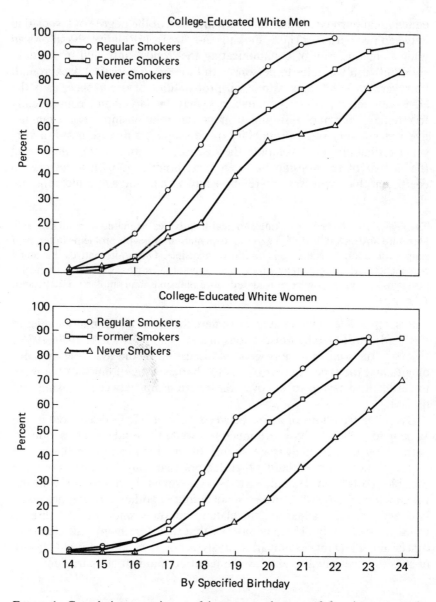

FIGURE 1. Cumulative experience of intercourse by age of first intercourse for college-educated white men and women in the United States who were regular smokers, former smokers, or never smokers. (*Note*. Data from National Individual Survey of Youth. Ohio State University, Center for Human Structure Research. Data extracted and graphed by Dr. Myron Johnson (personal communication, Jan, 1988.)

example, shows cumulative intercourse experience in college-educated white men and women; obviously, there are very large differences between regular smokers, quitters, and never smokers at age 20; for intance, 63% of women who were regular smokers had had intercourse but only 23% of women who had never smoked. Thus, if a correlation is found between smoking and cancer of the cervix, say, this association might be due entirely to the fact that women who are more sexually active are more likely to develop cancer of the cervix (Eysenck, 1980). To discover whether smoking has a separate effect, one would have to ascertain, and partial out statistically, the effects of a sexually active life-style. Given the large number of possible risk factors, such an exercise would be difficult, and certainly, the vast majority of reports do not attempt to rule out alternative hypotheses.

Perhaps more important than sexual activity are eating and drinking. The average smoker household, for instance, spends two to three times as much as the nonsmoker houshold on beer and 73% more on coffee. Equally, smoker households, relative to nonsmoker households, spend a larger share of their food dollars on products that are reportedly bad (red meat and eggs) and less on foods that are supposed to be good (cereals, fruits, and vegetables). (M. Johnston, personal communication, January, 1988.) This opens up the possibility that differences that allegedly are due to smoking (and passive smoking) may really be due to different drinking and eating patterns of different households. Certainly, no statistics that do not control for this (and many other) smoking-correlated factors can be taken very seriously.

An alternative method to multivariate analyses of this kind, which may be difficult or even impossible in view of the large number of correlated risk factors, is the intervention study, in which one variable is experimentally manipulated (e.g., smoking), and the effects are noted. It is because of the inherent methodological superiority of this method that the effects of quitting smoking are discussed in Chapter 2; the results, as mentioned, do not support the view that smoking exerts a strong influence on the development of cancer and CHD.

4
The Methodology of Epidemiological Studies of Smoking

What are the major arguments in favor of a close connection between smoking and disease, possibly interpretable in causal terms? The first argument, already considered to some extent, deals with the mortality ratios for different diseases, that is, figures purporting to demonstrate that smokers of a given age and sex die more frequently of a given disease than nonsmokers. The difference can be expressed as the "mortality ratio" (age-standardized mortality rate, or SMR), indicating the proportion of smokers to nonsmokers who are certified as having died of a particular disease. These ratios are usually in excess of 1.0 for a great variety of diseases, with the highest mortality ratio being that of cancer of the lung, followed by bronchitis and emphysema and cancer of the larynx and the oral cavity. Some mortality ratios, however, are below 1: for example, for cancer of the rectum, .90 (Kahn, 1966); colorectal cancer in women (.78 and .66 for women who smoked heavily, Hammond, 1966); and Parkinson's disease (.26, Kahn, 1966; .81 for an older group, Hammond, 1966). Eysenck (1987) gives a survey of the literature. He stresses that these figures should not be taken to indicate a beneficial effect of smoking, just as the positive mortality ratios for lung cancer and so on do not necessarily indicate the nefarious effect of smoking; the problem of inferring causation from correlation is, of course, too complex for such easy inferences.

The second argument often advanced is that when mortality ratios such as these refer to the position of a particular country at a particular time with respect to smoking and mortality, there appears to be a relationship between the crude male death rate for lung cancer and per capita consumption of cigarettes 20 years earlier, calculated over a number of countries; the time difference of 20 years is used because it is believed that smoking affects health only after lengthy periods of use.

A third argument is related to the fact that when mortality rates are examined by birth cohorts, it can be seen that most male and female cohorts, with increasing smoking prevalence, also have increasing age-specific mortality rates. In other words, the amount of smoking appears to correlate with the prevalence of lung cancer over time (dose–effect paradigm).

The fourth argument, already examined, relates to the alleged fact that quitting smoking will result in a lower mortality ratio, depending on the number of years since quitting smoking. These four arguments have been repeated time and again, and data also have been given apparently to support them. I have examined the data on cessation of smoking (Chapter 2) and shown that these in fact do not bear out the "orthodox" view but rather indicate that quitting smoking, when the proper controls are imposed on the study, has little or no effect on future CHD or cancer. Following is a consideration of the other points raised and the method-ological and statistical weaknesses that make the argument invalid.

First, it is necessary to mention one point that is often alleged to prove a direct causal relationship between smoking and oral carcinogenesis. Much effort has been spent in finding animal models that might be used to support this view, and researchers often claim that studies have succeeded in finding direct evidence. This, however, is not true. As the U.S. Surgeon General's report (1982) makes clear, "The useful animal model for the experimental study of all carcinogenesis has not been found. Cigarette smoke and cigarette smoke condensates generally fail to produce ma-lignancy when applied to the oral cavities of mice, rabbits or hamsters. Mechanical factors such as secretion of saliva interfere with the retention of carcinogenic agents" (p. 89). Thus, the statistical and epidemiological studies must bear the whole burden of the exercise; it is impermissible to quote animal experiments in this connection.

Quality of Epidemiological Data

Discussion of the epidemiological data may begin by stating the obvious, namely, that any conclusions that can be drawn from a statistical study of epidemiological data depend not only on the logic of the experimental design or the quality of the statistical analysis but even more crucially on the *quality of the actual data collected*. If the data themselves are highly unreliable, and in particular when they are biased, erroneous conclusions may be drawn even though methodology and statistical analysis appear impeccable. The data that epidemiologists mostly rely on usually are diag-noses made by a physician and recorded on the death certificate; data of this kind have been used in the official reports by the U.S. Surgeon General and the Royal College of Physicians, which have not seriously dealt with the question of misdiagnosis and reliability of data. Neither have these reports discussed the possibility of bias, which appears to be a very real danger in this field.

There has been a good deal of criticism of the use of statistics derived from diagnoses on death certificates; they have been generally considered to be inaccurate and unrealiable (J.H. Abramson, Sacks, & Cabana, 1971; Beadenkopf, Abrams, Daoud, & Marks, 1963; Briggs, 1975; Wells, 1923; Willis, 1967). Surveys by Britton (1974), Cameron & McGoogan, 1981), Gruver and Freis (1957), Hartveit (1979), Heasman and Lipworth (1966), and Waldron and Vickerstaff (1977) have given ample support to these criticisms. Britton (1974), for instance, found that the reported frequency of disagreements between clinical and autopsy diagnoses ranges from 6% to 65%! If we regard autopsies as completely reliable criteria (an assumption which, as will be discussed, is not entirely true), then clearly, the amount of inaccuracy in diagnoses is unacceptable for serious statistical work.

Some quotations may give a rough idea of the consensus in this area. Bauer and Robbins (1972) state that "our study indicates that accurate clinical diagnoses of cancer are as much a problem today as they were a half-century ago" (p. 1474). Abramson, Sacks, and Caban (1971) state that "the death certificate data had marked limitations as an indication of the presence of myocardial infarction, cerebrovascular disease, pulmonary embolisms or infarctions. . . . They gave a fairly accurate indication of the presence of malignant neoplasms but not of the specific sites or categories of neoplasms" (p. 430). And Britton (1974) concluded that "autopsies earlier did and still do reveal a considerable number of errors in clinical diagnoses. . . . There is no convincing sign that the rate of errors had diminished over the years" (p. 208). So much for the accuracy of the data on which the "orthodox" view is based.

As an example of the most carefully planned and conducted work in this field, let us consider the study by Cameron and McGoogan (1981). They reported a prospective study of 1,152 hospital autopsies, comparing these with death certification in each case. They were merely concerned with the *major* disease leading to death, as indicated by the physician completing the death certificate. They found that the main clinical diagnosis was confirmed in 703 out of 1,152 cases, or in 61%, leaving an error of 39%. This figure is not far removed from that observed by Britton (1974) in Sweden, where he found, in a careful, clinically controlled assessment, that main clinical diagnoses were confirmed in 57% of cases, leaving an error of 43%. Heasman and Lipworth (1966) and Waldron and Vickerstaff (1977) reported confirmed diagnoses in only 45% and 47.5%, respectively, leaving error rates of 55% and 52.5%. It is small surprise that Cameron and McGoogan (1981) concluded that, "In our experience, statistics from death certificates are so inaccurate that they are not suitable for use in research or planning" (p. 281). If this be true, then, clearly, all the statistical work supporting the received view is based on extremely uncertain foundations.

One other item of interest emerged from the Cameron and McGoogan (1981) study: a marked increase in the proportion of diagnostic discrepancies with increasing age of the subjects. For subjects less than 45 years of age, diagnoses were correct in 78%, but thereafter, they fell off in a step-like manner with each succeeding decade until, for subjects over 75 years, fewer than half were confirmed. This has particular relevance to the incidence of lung cancer, because this, of course, occurs mainly in older men and women.

It is of interest to look specifically at data for neoplasms and for CHD diagnoses, because errors in these are of special relevance to the topic of this book. Cancer of the bronchus/lung was correctly diagnosed in 88 cases and wrongly diagnosed in 61 cases; thus, the error rate is about the same as for all diseases. Bauer and Robbins (1972) looked at autopsies on 2,734 cancer patients and found that 26% had clinically undiagnosed cancer; in a further 14%, the condition was incompletely diagnosed, that is, cancer was suspected, but its primary site was not known or was wrongly identified. Cameron and McGoogan (1981) conclude their comments on neoplasms by stating, "Carcinoma of bronchus was the most common neoplasm in our series and provided the largest group of misdiagnoses" (p. 294).

Turning now to cardiorespiratory conditions, for acute myocardial infarct, agreement occurs in 198 cases, and disagreement in 109 cases— again, an unacceptable level of error of diagnoses. Cerebrovascular disease scored an agreement in 129 cases and disagreement in 118 cases, with an error rate of almost 50%. "The most common problem of differential diagnosis appeared to be in distinguishing it from cardiovascular disease," Cameron and McGoogan (1981) stated (p. 293). Hartveit (1979), Heasman and Lipworth (1966), and Kagan Katsuki, Sternley, and Venecek (1967) also found a large amount of overdiagnosis and underdiagnosis of cerebrovascular disease.

Detection Bias

When diagnoses are as unreliable as they have been found to be in the case of lung cancer and CHD, one must be particularly concerned about the phenomenon of "detection bias," that is, the tendency of the physician to diagnose "smoking related diseases" in smokers rather than in non-smokers. Feinstein and Wells (1974) have published data to show that such detection bias is a reality and might easily lead to false conclusions in the absence of careful necropsy examinations of the causes of death. Detection bias undoubtedly contributes part of the high mortality ratios for lung cancer often reported and should be carefully excluded in any study purporting to have scientific validity.

Feinstein and Wells (1974) looked at data concerning 654 patients who were diagnosed after necropsy as having died of lung cancer. In this series, they studied the relationship between the rate of nondiagnosis during life and the amount of antecedent cigarette smoking. In patients whose history of cigarette smoking was unknown, this nondiagnosis rate was 37%. The rate of nondiagnosis then portrays a distinctive downward gradient, falling from 38% undetected among noncigarette smokers, to 20% among the light smokers, 14% in the moderate, and 10% and 11%, respectively, in the heavy and extreme smokers. "The data therefore suggested that the more patients smoke, the more likely they were to have the lung cancer detected during life," stated Feinstein and Wells (1974, p. 185).

Feinstein and Wells (1974) also investigated how this premortem detection gradient was related to the intensity of diagnostic examinations received during life by patients in their entire series, which included 677 cases that were diagnosed during life but received no necropsy. The authors used for this purpose the Papanicolaou cytologic examination (or pap smear) of the sputum. Because this test had not been obtained by all of their patients, its solicitation might have been affected by diverse factors, including the patient's smoking history. They therefore examined the pap smear research rate, and the results are in agreement with this hypothesis. The test was requested more frequently in smokers than in nonsmokers. Statistical tests showed that the trend was very highly significant. Detection bias was consequently found to be distinctly related to the amount of cigarette smoking.

Space does not permit discussion of the other analyses by Feinstein and Wells, which tend to support the following general conclusion:

Cigarette smoking may contribute more to the diagnosis of lung cancer than it does to producing the disease itself.... It seems important to recall that in epidemiologic surveys of causes of disease, the investigators get data about the occurrence of diagnoses not the occurrence of diseases, and that the rates of diagnosis may be affected by bias in the way that doctors order and deploy the available diagnostic technology. (Feinstein & Wells, 1974, p. 184)

Taken together with the general unreliability of diagnoses of lung cancer, these findings (Feinstein & Wells, 1974) make it doubly improbable that the observed diagnostic data that furnish the foundations for epidemiological studies can be taken seriously by scientific investigators. More research is urgently required on the actual unreliability of diagnoses, as well as on "detection bias"; if reliable data on these two points were available, then statistical corrections might be made to the published data on the relationship between smoking and lung cancer. Without such data, all conclusions clearly are based on very unfirm foundations indeed.

Is Lung Cancer?

What light do these considerations throw on the problem of the apparent rapid rise in lung cancer over the years? This is copiously illustrated in the report of the U.S. Surgeon General, together with the rise, 20 years previously, of cigarette consumption; it will be remembered that this temporal correlation is one of the major arguments put forward by epidemiologists in favor of the "orthodox" view. At the same time, this apparent rise presents great difficulties for those who, like Burch (1976) and myself (Eysenck, 1986), argue in favor of theories of the conception and development of carcinomas that are based on genetic hypotheses and partly disregard the role of external carcinogens. It is implausible to argue that there have been genetic changes of such a size and nature as to cause such manifold increases in the occurrence of lung cancer, and consequently, the argument for the causal effects of environmental changes, air pollution, and cigarette smoking, for example, must be taken seriously. An alternative suggestion is that the increase in deaths diagnosed as lung cancer has been due to improvements in diagnostic techniques and is therefore more apparent than real. This argument has been put forward by Rigdon and Kirchoff (1953), who concluded that claims of genuine increase in the frequency of lung cancer were "open to question." Willis (1967), after an extensive review of the literature, concluded, "It is not possible either to affirm or to deny that there has been a real increase" (p. 187). Similarly, Feinstein (1988) concluded his historical discussion by stating that diagnostic changes have played the most important role in the increase in death rate from lung cancer. Burch (1976) cites much evidence to support this view.

It seems certain that, in the first years of the century, lung cancer was considerably underdiagnosed. Sehrt (1904) described 178 cases of lung cancer discovered at necropsy, only six of which had been recognized during life. If we take this ratio of 172 failures to diagnose lung cancer as compared with six successful diagnoses of lung cancer and argue that with our modern techniques all or most of the 178 cases of lung cancer would have been so diagnosed, then it seems quite reasonable to assume that much if not all of the apparent increase in deaths from lung cancer may have been due to improvements in diagnostic techniques.

The evidence suggests that at present there is a considerable over-diagnosis of lung cancer, and the question arises: What causes false-positive diagnoses? Rosenblatt (1974) has suggested that in the post-1930 period, false-positive clinical diagnoses of lung cancer often were due to metastases in the lung from primary locations at many different sites. He too believed that the very great increase in recorded lung cancer deaths over the past 30 years was not due to an extrinsic carcinogen but resulted from the use of new diagnostic techniques, in particular, radiology, bronchoscopy, sputum examination, and surgery. He further suggested that the great interest in lung cancer stimulated by the theory that it might be due to somking had produced a tendency to overdiagnose this particular disorder, and Smithers (1953) discovered that even specialists in thoracic diseases were guilty of a large proportion of false-positive diagnoses from 1944 to 1950.

Rosenblatt, Teng, Kerpe, and Beck (1971) supported this argument by showing that, at the Doctors' Hospital in New York, clinical diagnosis of lung cancer was more than twice as frequent as diagnosis following necropsy. Carcinoma of the lung was the only neoplasma found to be greatly overdiagnosed clinically and in which no unsuspected cases were found at necropsy. Primary lung cancer had been simulated by pulmonary metastases from carcinoma of the pancreas, kidney, stomach, breast, and thyroid, and by malignant melanoma. Burch (1976) makes the following interesting comment:

It is of great interest that the 5.5% of lung cancers found in this recent New York necropsy series of malignancy is *lower* than a proportion found amongst several necropsy series from Austria, Germany and the U.S. published at the end of the 19th and beginning of the 20th century. In five subseries in which necropsy findings were the main basis of diagnosis, lung cancer diagnosis ranged from 8.3% to 11.5% of all cancers (p. 329).

This finding must throw doubt on the alleged increase in lung cancer.

The problem of metastasis to the lung being erroneously diagnosed as lung cancer is emphasized by a study reported by Burch (1978). He found that a total of 747 primary lung cancers was recorded in a large-scale postmortem study of the anatomical distribution of metastases in Swedish cancer cases but some 2,079 metastases to the lung from primary sites outside the lung! Burch gives many other instances, and it is difficult not to agree with him when he concludes, "There can be no doubt . . . that diagnostic artefacts have contributed massively to the secular increases in recorded deaths rates from lung cancer. . . . The beginning of the century was characterized by a severe under-diagnosis, especially above the age of 40 years" (p. 458).

In this discussion, I have assumed that autopsies normally will constitute a completely reliable criterion. However, it is fairly optimistic to imagine that diagnoses, even when based on autopsies, can be relied on to give a true picture of the actual condition that caused death. An editorial ("Medical Charities and Prevention," 1971) in the *Annals of Thoracic Surgery* pointed out that "The most experienced pathologists often disagree on classification of these tumours, and differential criteria are poorly defined." Large bodies of data are available to indicate that the reliability of medical diagnosis using pathological material relevant to respiratory diseases is well below what would be regarded as acceptable in psychological tests (see Kern, Jones, & Chapman, 1968; McCarthy & Widmer, 1974; Reid & Rose, 1964; Stebbings, 1971; Thurlbeck et al., 1968; Wilson & Burke, 1957; Yesner, Selfman, & Feinstein, 1973).

Autopsies, while greatly superior to deathbed diagnoses, are obviously still unreliable, in that different experts have different views. Such unreliability makes validity suspect, although it would be difficult to give a numerical assessment of the degree of unreliability or the lack of validity in these data.

The difficulties introduced by errors in the certification of the cause of death make it desirable to study trends in *overall* mortality, rather than mortality that is due to specific diseases. Doll and Peto (1976) conducted a large-scale study of this kind and concluded that "much of the excess mortality in cigarette smokers could be attributed with certainty to the habit." Burch (1978) examined this conclusion and carried out a large-scale statistical analysis of smoking and mortality in England and Wales from 1950 to 1976, calculating percentage changes in sex- and age-specific death rates for all causes of death in England and Wales by 3-year periods. These changes in death rates were compared with corresponding trends and sex- and age-specific "constant tar" and "current" cigarette consumption in the United Kingdom. He concluded that "No obvious cause-and-effect relation can be discerned" (Burch, 1978, p. 87). As Burch points out, the main problem is to explain the fairly consistent *decrease* in death rates in both sexes and all age group during periods when cigarette consumption was either rising or falling. "The trends failed to support the hypothesis that smoking influenced mortality," he states (p. 87). Burch concluded:

This paper has shown that secular trends in overall mortality in England and Wales give no consistent indication that they were appreciably influenced by changes in cigarette consumption . . . on scientific grounds there can be little doubt that the conclusions drawn by the Royal College of Physicians (1971), Doll and Peto (1976), and the Surgeon-General of the United States (1979) about the lethality of smoking are precipitate and unwarranted. (p. 102)

In addition to the uncertain state of the death certificate diagnosis, there is another serious directional error in the ascertainment of number of cigarettes smoked. In one of the unpublished Grossarth-Maticek and Eysenck studies, we looked at the accuracy of such statements, better ways of getting accurate statements, and directionality of errors. In the first study, we had probands estimate the number of cigarettes smoked; we also had close relatives (usually the spouse) make an analogous estimate. Finally, we instructed probands to keep a 7-day journal, noting down each cigarette smoked and the occasion. We found for 136 participants that the self-estimate was 12 cigarettes per day. Relatives estimated 18; the journal disclosed 19. The proband's own estimate was a 50% underestimate.

In this study, a personality inventory, to be described later, was given after the estimate was made. We advanced the hypothesis that if the inventory was administered first, it would make the proband more likely to give truthful answers. In the matched group of 136 smoking, the three estimates agreed very well: own estimate 17, relative's estimate 16, journal record 18. In our own work, to be described, this second method has been followed.

This degree of inaccuracy is particularly troublesome if it is directional, that is, if cancer-prone probands were to overestimate and not-prone probands were to underestimate the number of cigarettes smoked. In a group of 128 cancer-prone probands, ascertained on the basis of a personality inventory, as described in Chapter 6, the self-estimation averaged 17, relative's estimation averaged 16, and the journal averaged 15. The other personality types investigated showed underestimations of between 2 and 18 cigarettes per day, instead of the overestimation of 2 cigarettes of the cancer-prone probands. This tendency, in general, would greatly exaggerate the statistical correlation between cancer and smoking. Clearly, careful experimenters would look at sources of error of this kind and try to eliminate them; this has not happened in the great majority of studies examined.

I have devoted a considerable amount of space to a discussion of the reliability of the data and possible biases in the data, because all conclusions in science depend absolutely on the quality of the data. When the data are as poor as those used by epidemiologists to establish a relationship between smoking and cancer, and smoking and CHD, then a detailed demonstration of the unreliability and invalidity of the data is imperative. It is noteworthy that those who maintain the "orthodox" view seldom argue the case; they accept faulty data without any query and without answering the critics who draw attention to these fundamental faults.

Another vital criticism of the orthodox view relates to an argument in the U.S. Surgeon General's (1982) report to the effect that "The relative risk ratio measures the strength of an association and provides an evaluation of the importance of that factor in the production of a disease" (p. 17). Such a statement contravenes the logic of epidemiological inquiry and takes for granted that which is to be proved; clearly, the risk ratio only provides an evaluation of the importance of the factor in the production of the disease once it has been proved that there is a causal relationship! The strength and consistency of the association cannot be used to prove a causal relationship. However, the *absence* of a consistency in the strength of the association certainly can be used to throw doubt on the causal implications. From the hypothesis of the universal causal effects of smoking on lung cancer, similar or identical risk ratios should be found, say, in Oriental and white populations. This, however, is not so (Eysenck, 1980, 1986).

Race and Sex in Bronchial Carcinoma

Mortality risks in the dominantly white populations cluster around an average mortality rate of about 10, ranging from 7.0 to 14.2. Values in Mongoloid populations, however, are very different. In Japan, the value is 3.8; for Chinese residents in Singapore, it is 3.8 also (McLennan et al., 1977). In Northern Thailand, a value of 1.6 has been reported by Simarak, de Jong, Breslow, and Dahl (1977), that is not significantly different from unity, showing an effect of smoking. Similarly, a risk ratio of 1.57 has been reported from Mainland China. For women, the incidence of lung cancer in the Chinese in Hong Kong was reported as only 1.74 by Chan, Colbourne, Fung, and Ho (1979). In Hawaii, relative risk ratios of 10.5, 4.9, and 1.8, respectively, were found for women of Hawaiian, Japanese, and Chinese origin; this aligns the Hawaiian women with the white mortality ratios and contrasts them with the Japanese and Chinese women studied (Hinds et al., 1981). Many other studies can be quoted to substantiate the existence of important racial differences in risk ratios between white and oriental groups, particularly women. Examples are studies by Leung (1977), Gao, Blot, Zheng, Franmini and Hsu (1988), and Green and Art (1982); see also the book on "Geographical Pathology in Cancer Epidemiology" by Grundmann, Clemmesen and Muir (1982). It is difficult to account for these very large differences in mortality ratios between white and Oriental groups in terms of the orthodox view; it is much more natural to appeal to genetic causes in this context.

Many other facts have been adduced to support this view Eysenck (1965, 1980). The important work of Belcher (1971) has reported on worldwide differences in the sex ratio of bronchial carcinoma. The ratio of men affected, as compared with women, varies widely from one part of the world to another. In Nigeria, for instance, the incidence is actually higher among the women than among the men, whereas in Holland, it is over 13 times higher in men as compared with women. There is no relationship between the sex ratio and the total tobacco consumption in different countries, nor is the different age structure of the different populations responsible. Belcher concludes that "there is a genetic factor in the aetiology of bronchial carcinoma" (p. 220). All these data are not interpretable in terms of the orthodox view and throw much doubt on its value in interpreting the observed facts.

Another argument made much use of by the U.S. Surgeon General and the Royal College of Physicians is an alleged "dose–response" relationship. As the Surgeon General's report states: "Important to the strength as well as to the coherence of the association, is the presence of the dosage-response phenomenon in which a positive gradient between the degree of exposure to the agent and incidence or mortality rates of the disease can be demonstrated" (p. 17).

Such a dose–response relationship, however would also be predicted from other hypotheses, as Burch (1983) has pointed out:

To take the simplest postulates, smokers can be divided into two categories, social and habituated. Social smokers tend to be light smokers and could quit readily; habituated, genetically-predisposed smokers, tend to be heavy smokers. Hence, in any group of light smokers, social smokers will predominate and the association with lung cancer will be relatively weak; in any group of heavy smokers, habituated, genetically-predisposed smokers will predominate and the association with lung cancer will be strong. An apparent "dose–response" relation will be observed." (p. 826)

Dose-Response Relationships?

The causal hypothesis, in its pure form, would predict the same response from the same "dose" in different populations; the genetic hypothesis, which assumes that the association between smoking and lung cancer depends on the strength of the associations between patients' presenting genotypes, rather than on smoking levels, would predict some correlations, though not necessarily very high ones, between national mortality and national smoking levels. The observed relationship between national mortality from lung cancer and national cigarette consumption is not very strong. An example of discordance is the age-standardized mortality from lung cancer in Finnish men in 1960 to 1961, which was about double that in U.S. white men, whereas cigarette consumption in 1950 in Finland was about half that in the United States (Burch, 1976). There are many other anomalies of this kind, as the perusal of the report will show; Burch (1983) has pointed out: "The pure causal hypothesis might, by this test alone, appear to be untenable. The existence of the weak correlation between national rates of mortality and smoking is consistent with the causal component but it is also consistent with the pure constitutional hypothesis and no causal action" (p. 826).

Passey (1961) has thrown doubt on the existence of a proper dose–response relationship within a given population. As he points out, "Nowhere has it been claimed that the heavy smoker is stricken with cancer earlier than the light smoker. If lung cancer in smokers is the result of direct carcinogenic action, one would certainly expect this to happen; for experiment has shown beyond question that a potent carcinogen induces tumours early" (p. 110). Passey next examined the smoking history of 499 men with lung cancer, grouping the cases according to the number of cigarettes smoked. He gives a table that shows the following:

The amount smoked makes no appreciable difference to the mean age at which the person first reported to the clinic. The light smokers is afflicted with lung cancer at the same age as a heavy smoker. This is a surprising observation. The mean age at which smoking was started was 17; the average amount smoked daily was 23 cigarettes; the mean age at which the patient presented at the clinic was 57 years . . . the mean smoking period was some 40 years. (p. 109)

Nor was it true, as might be said, that the youngest of these patients with lung cancer might have smoked particularly heavily or that the eldest had survived because they were specially moderate smokers:

The amount smoked daily by old and young is not dissimilar. Yet the oldest patient had smoked for some 50 years longer than the youngest patient—this represents well over a quarter of a million more cigarettes. These figures suggest that there is no relation between the amount smoked daily and the age of onset of lung cancer. (Passey, 1961, p. 111)

Pike and Doll (1965) replicated Passey's findings from their sample of British doctors. They concluded that "Neither the amount smoked nor the age of starting made any substantial difference to the average age of onset of the disease" (p. 667), and these conclusions were also found valid for the "life-span" average under the conditions in which lung cancer is produced in humans.

The Same Paradoxes

Last but not least in discussing the strength of the association, one must consider the paradox presented by mortality ratios as related to degree of inhalation. On the orthodox view, it would be expected that inhalation would give much higher mortality ratios, for equal amounts amoked, than would lack of inhalation. Fisher (1959) analyzed retrospective data of disease by daily rate of smoking; inhalers had a paradoxically lower risk of lung cancer than noninhalers. Doll and Peto (1976), in a 20-year follow-up of British male doctors, standardized for age and amount smoked (in nine groups) found that the overall risk of lung cancer in inhalers was 84% of that of noninhalers. A thorough discussion of the evidence is given by Eysenck (1980).

Stolley (in press) has argued, on the basis of more recent work, that Fischer was wrong in suggesting that inhaling actually protected the smoker, and he undoubtedly exaggerated the import of a small difference not found in later work; even so, the impact of inhaling is not what we would have expected theoretically.

Much is made by adherents of the orthodox view of the temporal congruence between increases in smoking and increases in lung cancer. The alleged increase in the incidence of lung cancer has been discussed here, and as mentioned, the evidence does not really support any such increase but rather suggests that changes in diagnostic methods enable identification of lung cancer more readily (and perhaps too readily, considering the overdiagnosis mentioned previously).

Of particular interest is the temporal relationship observed in the differential patterns for males and females. In the United Kingdom, a sharp increase in cigarette consumption occurred among women about 30 years after it occurred among men. Burch (1976, 1983), however, has shown:

When rise in recorded mortality from lung cancer is studied in detail, it is seen that the temporal pattern of increments, from one five-year period to the next, is remarkably synchronous in the two sexes from the beginning of the century to 1955 and then from 1965 onwards. It follows that the main causes of the recorded increases in both sexes were also synchronous in both sexes and therefore could not have been cigarette smoking. (1983, p. 828)

Thus, what is claimed to be one of the strongest proofs for the received view turns out, on detailed examination, to be a strong argument against that view.

One other example of the numerous inconsistencies in the way of temporal relationships must suffice. Guberan (1979) has demonstrated a surprising decline of cardiovascular mortalities in Switzerland from 1951 to 1976, in spite of *increasing* smoking by women and roughly stationary smoking rates in men. Guberan also reported a 20% rise in consumption of animal fats; yet age-standardized death rates for all diseases of the circulatory system decreased by 22% in men and by 43% in women. These results are difficult to assimilate for adherents of the orthodox view.

As an example of the complexity of the issues encountered by epidemiologists, consider laryngeal cancer. Rothman, Cann, Flanders, and Fried (1980) demonstrate a linear regression of age-standardized mortality from laryngeal cancer on number of cigarettes smoked daily (p. 201). Yet Curwen, Kanaway, and Kanaway (1954) and McMichael (1978) failed to discover the expected dramatic upsurge of such cancer in recent years, to parallel the (alleged) dramatic increase in lung cancer! Perhaps methods of diagnosis for laryngeal cancer have not shown the great improvement that methods of diagnosis for lung cancer have enjoyed.

One must conclude that the study of the temporal relationship of the association between cigarette smoking and cancer is vitiated by the poor quality of the data, but that does not offer any support for the orthodox view.

Long-Term Studies

Do we find any support in long-term studies, which would be the ideal testing ground for causal theories? Vaillant and Vaillant (1990) have recently reported on a 45-year follow-up study of former Harvard University sophomores, in which they looked at a large number of possible risk factors for mental and physical health, including smoking. Smoking did correlate with physical health ($r = -.13$), but at a level too low to be of much practical significance. Psychosocial factors proved much more predictive. Thus, childhood strengths ($r = .26$) and emotional closeness to siblings ($r = .18$), maturity of defenses ($r = .19$), and good psychosocial adjustment at age 47 ($r = .19$) were more predictive, and "the most significant predictor of both physical and mental ill health at age 65 was mood-altering drug use before age 50" (Vaillant & Vaillant, p. 34)—itself, of course, highly correlated with psychosocial factors like depression ($r = -.36$). This variable is thus many times more predictive of ill health than smoking. And, as one might have expected, in their multivariate analysis (p. 35), smoking disappears altogether, and the variables that predict physical health are psychosocial, genetic, exercise, and drug taking (alcohol and mood-altering drugs before age 50). Again, one should not deny that smoking has any deleterious effects on health, but the study suggests that it should be viewed as one of many risk factors and far from the most important.

Passive Smoking

This chapter has examined some of the criticisms of the methodology and the data used to establish the orthodox view; a much more detailed account has been given elsewhere (Eysenck, 1980, 1986). I have not yet extended the review to the issue of "passive" smoking; the notion that passive smoking can cause disease has been criticized on methodological and statistical grounds by Aviado (1986), and nothing in the recent literature alters his verdict:

That there is no substantial evidence to support the view that exposure to environmental tobacco smoking presents a significant health hazard to the non-smoker. After a detailed consideration of the circulatory and respiratory diseases studies, it is concluded that there are inadequate data on which to base the conclusion that exposure to environmental tobacco smoke causes such diseases. Consequently, in this author's view, non-smokers should not use claims of adverse health effects as justification for not interacting with smokers in society. (Aviado, 1986, p. 158)

Is this conclusion faulted by more recent evidence? The report of the National Health and Medical Research Council (NHMRC) of Australia (1987) is not intemperate in its conclusions. They note:

In several important areas, there is insufficient scientific evidence yet available. In particular: (1) the effect on lung function of acute exposure to passive smoke in healthy individuals appears not to be substantial nor is the evidence consistent; (2) few data are available regarding the effects upon both the upper and lower respiratory tracts of chronic passive smoking in healthy individuals; and (3) there are no data on the effects of passive smoking during childhood on subsequent lung function in adulthood (p. 44)

With regard to lung cancer, they say that there is mounting epidemiological evidence that passive smoking *may* increase the risk of occurrence of lung cancer but they note "limitations in the amount of data available" and "research difficulties in making satisfactory estimations of individual exposure;" all this is perfectly reasonable. They also note that "there is very limited evidence available about the cardiovascular effects of passive smoking." (p. 44.) The council finally "acknowledge[s] that further research is necessary to confirm and elaborate the effects of passive smoking upon health" (p. 45).

The report of the U.S. Surgeon General (1989) is much more intemperate. Thus, it is asserted that "it is cerain that a substantial proportion of the lung cancers that occur in non-smokers are due to ETS [environmental tobacco smoke] exposure"; the report admits, though, that "more complete data on the dose and variability of smoke exposure in the non-smoking U.S. population will be needed before a quantitative estimate of the number of such cancers can be made" (p. X). Regarding the relationship between ETS and cancers other than lung cancer and cardiovascular disease, the report states that "further research in these areas will be required to determine whether an association exists between ETS exposure and an increased risk of developing those diseases" (p. XI).

On what sort of evidence is all this based? As the Australian report states, the conclusions depend on "observing empirical associations between reported individual smoking habits and the occurrence of cancer. Such observations are made in either cohort (prospective) studies or case-control (retrospective) studies" (NHMRC, 1987, p. 27.) Many difficulties and problematical assumptions are involved in this process. As the authors of the U.S. Surgeon General's report (1989) point out, "the quantification of the risks associated with involuntary smoking . . . is dependent on a number of factors on which only a limited amount of data are currently available" (p. 96). The first such factor noted is the absolute magnitude of the lung cancer risk associated with involuntary smoking; the studies cited in the report do not contain a zero-exposure group. "The magnitude of the difference in tobacco smoke exposure between groups identified by spousal smoking habits may vary from study to study; this variation may partially explain the differences in risk estimates among the studies" (p. 96).

The second factor noted is the lack of suitable data on the dose and distribution of exposure to ETS in the population. "The studies that have been performed have attempted to identify groups with different exposures, but little is known about the magnitude of the exposures that occur in different segments of the U.S. population or about the variability of exposure with time of day or seasons of the year" (U.S. Surgeon General, 1989, p. 96). In other words, fundamental and basic facts are not known.

Of 13 studies cited in the U.S. Surgeon General's report (1989), 7 give insignificant results; the fact that so few give statistically significant results makes the report plead for the use of one-tail tests, in order to boost significance by inadmissible means—one is to assume what one is trying to prove! They argue that "the lack of statistical significance in all studies should not invalidate the positive significant associations for involuntary smoking that have been observed" (p. 97). But such a conclusion, of course, depends on the adequacy of the methodology of these studies.

The report notes several "serious criticisms," such as the misclassification of the active smoking status of the subjects, "which can produce an apparent increased risk with involuntary smoking" (U.S. Surgeon General, 1989, p. 101). The report also notes that "it is likely to result in differential misclassification because spouses tend to have similar smoking habits" (p. 101). "Misclassification of the lung as the primary site and the lack of pathological confirmation are repeated concerns" (p. 101). "Misclassification of exposure to ETS cannot be dismissed, since an index based solely on the smoking habits of a current spouse may not be indicative of past exposure, cumulative exposure, or the relevant dose to the respiratory tract" (p. 101). It is admitted that "the magnitude of risks associated with involuntary smoking exposure is uncertain" (p. 101). These are some of the criticisms voiced in the report; it does not seem reasonable to base any far-reaching conclusions on such doubtful data.

But worse still, the authors (U.S. Surgeon General, 1989) do not consider at all many of the cogent criticisms made of the "smoking causes cancer" literature, which apply with special force to ETS exposure. No attention is paid to the synergistic interaction of risk factors or the impermissible use of the concept of "cause" in the context of complex interrelations. Very doubtful and admittedly unquantifiable risk ratios become "substantial proportions" in the summary of the Surgeon General. No allowance is made for other risk factors, such as drinking, air pollution, stress, diet, and so on, whether correlated with smoking or not. To give but one simple example, if people smoke in part because they are under stress, then it seems likely that their spouses also will be under stress; as will be discussed, stress is a strong risk factor for lung cancer and may mediate the (at best weak) association between ETS exposure and lung cancer. Hundreds of such alternative possibilities suggest themselves, but none are mentioned or investigated by the authors of the report. Science advances by a considertion of plausible alternative hypotheses not by complete disregard of explanations that may conflict with assumed dogma.

Finally, consider the validity of the statistics employed. The most widely quoted results favoring an association between passive smoking and lung cancer are those of Hirayama (1981a) and Trichopolous, Kalondidi, Sparrow, and MacMahon (1981). As regards the first of these, Mantel (1981) provided a detailed criticism of the statistics, to which Hirayama (1981b) failed to respond properly but added some new information. Lee (1981) further showed that Hirayama's 11 printed confidence intervals were all in error by factors of up to 1,000%, errors later acknowledged by Hirayama (1981b). The work of Trichopolous et al. (1981, 1983) has also been shown to be faulty, as pointed out by Heller (1983). Trichopolous (1984) excused this as a "typing error"—a rather causal response to a serious criticism of his principal conclusions!

The most recent study (Janerich, et al., 1990), concluding that "the evidence we report lends further support to the observation that passive smoking may increase the risk of subsequent lung cancer" (p. 636), may be useful in demonstrating the nonobjective nature of the argument, and in particular (a) the neglect of negative outcomes, (b) the refusal to consider alternative hypotheses, and (c) a neglect of elementary statistical principles. In this study, individually matched pairs (lung cancer patient vs. healthy control) were compared with respect to exposure to cigarette smoke. For overall exposure, "no clear dose–response relationship is evident" (p. 633), suggesting no overall effect. For exposure in childhood and adolescence, there is an overall effect. For smoking by the spouse, the most widely used measure, "there was little evidence of a trend according to amount of exposure" (p. 634). Exposure in the workplace indicated "no evidence of an adverse effect of environmental tobacco smoke" (p. 634). Finally, "our analysis of exposure in social settings . . . showed a statistically significant *inverse* association between environmental tobacco smoke and lung cancer" (Janerich et al., 1990, p. 634) (emphasis added).

What would a proper summary of this work be? It would stress (a) the lack of overall effect, showing no clear dose–response relationship; (b) the negative health effects of childhood and adolescent passive smoking contrasted with the positive health effects of social smoking: and (c) the lack of effect of workplace or spouse smoking. The authors concentrate on the one (out of four) negatively significant result, forgetting that statistical significance for one selected test out of four cannot be calculated as if this were the only test done and attempt to explain it by suggesting that during childhood and adolescence probands are more likely to be responsive to passive smoking, although "we know of no specific mechanism that would explain our findings" (p. 634). In other words, the "explanation" is purely ad hoc, and adds nothing to the alleged findings. They fail to discuss the fact that "the difference in the magnitude of the effect between exposure during childhood and adolescence and exposure during adulthood did not achieve statistical significance" (p. 634), a finding that would seem to disprove their own hypothesis.

Can one explain the "unexpected" protective effect of exposure to social smoking? A likely hypothesis would suggest that extraverted personality traits seem to protect against cancer and that cancer-prone individuals, as discussed in Chapters 6 and 7, have personality traits usually associated with introversion (Eysenck, 1990b). Extraverted people, however, are more likely than introverted ones to attend social functions and to be exposed to cigarette smoke. The hypothesis would explain the alleged protective function of social smoking as an artifact, which is due to personality characteristics shared by socially active persons and non–cancer-prone persons. The failure of Janerich et al, (1990) to take into account any risk factors other than smoking accounts for their failure to explain their own findings.

Finally, note that the logic of their argument should lead them to recommend exposure to social passive smoking as a potent protective method. If one is to take seriously epidemiological studies of this type and base recommendations on them, one should surely be less selective in one's conclusions and recommendations and stress findings incompatible with established theory.

One must conclude that, admittedly, little, if any, evidence links cancer or CHD with ETS exposure. For lung cancer, some published studies produce evidence of a statistically significant correlation (6 out of a total of 13), with a majority failing to produce such a correlation. The report (U.S. Surgeon General, 1989) recognizes serious criticisms of the work done, criticisms that seem to invalidate any positive conclusions. The report fails to deal with even more serious criticisms, including the impropriety of interpreting (doubtful) statistical associations in causal terms. One must conclude that Aviado's (1986) summary has not been overturned by the most recent evidence and that proof is still lacking concerning the adverse effects of passive smoking in cancer and CHD.

5
The Causes of Smoking: Needs or Addiction?

An important part of the orthodox view is that smoking is addictive, and hence that nicotine joins the addictive drugs such as heroin, LSD, and so on. A recent report of the U.S. Surgeon General (1988), "Nicotine Addiction," contains the following major conclusions:

1. Cigarettes and other forms of tobacco are addicting.
2. Nicotine is a drug in tobacco that causes addiction.
3. The pharmacologic and behavioral processes that determine tobacco addiction are similar to those that determine addiction to drugs such as heroin and cocaine. (p. 9)

Is it true that nicotine is an addictive drug, or is an alternative hypothesis more likely, namely, that nicotine has effects on human beings that fulfill certain needs, just as food satisfies the need caused by hunger and drink serves the need caused by thirst? This is an important debate, particularly, because it will be seen to lead into the question of personality as related to smoking, and smoking related diseases. A detailed account of the arguments has been given by Warburton (1985), who discusses the many meanings of the term *addiction* and also looks at the question raised by the U.S. Surgeon General in a detailed examination of the evidence (Warburton, 1989). As Warburton points out, originally, the term *addiction* was used for any strong inclination for any kind of conduct, good or bad. It is only recently that certain patterns of drug use have been labeled as addictions, and today, *addiction* is often used to imply an undesirable, and usually an illegal, use of drugs. In the same way, the noun *addict* has lost its denotative meaning of people engaged in certain habits and has become a stigmatizing label, implying someone with a disease.

Alcoholics and drug users in the past were regarded as morally depraved, but by the end of the 19th century, they were regarded as diseased (Berridge & Edwards, 1987). The disease concept of drug use carries with it the implication that the addict has some "physiological addiction mechanism," so that the person is at the mercy of physiological cravings. Similarly, relapse is a symptom of the reemerging disease. Other authors regard drug use as a type of mental disease, a lack of willpower, thus, linking notions of moral, psychological, and physiological pathology in the concept of addiction.

Definition of Addiction

As Warburton (1989) points out, the U.S. Surgeon General (1988) has produced lists of criteria for defining nicotine use as an "addiction" that depend on argument by analogy. Such arguments are dangerous; they may be used to suggest a conclusion, but they cannot establish it. Warburton argues that the U.S. Surgeon General has ignored the discrepancies in his argument in his enthusiasm to find criteria to compare nicotine users with heroin and cocaine users. The U.S. Surgeon General suggests three primary criteria. The first of these is that the drug has psychoactive effects. This is a novel criterion, not normally used in this field of substance use; it is supported by the U.S. Surgeon General's statement that "to distinguish drug dependence from habitual behaviors not involving drugs, it must be demonstrated that a drug with psychoactive (mood altering) effects in the brain enters the blood-stream" (pp. 7–8). As Warburton points out, this criterion is trivial. Entering the blood stream does not define psychoactivity; the important issue for the Surgeon General's argument is whether the actions of nicotine are like those of cocaine and the opiates. Certainly, both heroin, cocaine, and nicotine are psychoactive, but they are very different in their effects. Heroin induces euphoria, but it also impairs performance, and cocaine impairs judgment; nicotine, on the other hand, improves performance, renders the user more alert, increases efficiency of performance, and reduces anxiety (Warburton, Revell, & Walter, 1988). As Pomerleau and Pomerleau (1984) state: "In contrast to drugs of abuse, nicotine from smoking is not only compatible with work but actually facilitates performance of certain kinds of tasks" (p. 510). Thus, in terms of psychoactive drug use, nicotine has a behavioral mode of action quite different from heroin and cocaine.

The second major criterion adduced by the U.S. Surgeon General relates to drug-reinforced behavior, which means "the pharmacological activity of the drug is sufficiently rewarding to maintain self-administration." With drugs such as heroin and cocaine, rats and monkeys can be readily trained to press a lever to obtain an injection, but this is not so with nicotine. It is difficult to train monkeys to lever press for nicotine, and the pattern of administration bears no relation to human smoking.

The whole argumemt seems beside the point. According to the report: "Addicting drugse often provide . . . benefit or otherwise useful effect; these effects may also contribute to the compulsive nature of drug use" (p. 250). What this statement seems to mean is that if something is beneficial, it can be addicting! This would suggest that food and sex are "addictive"!

The third major criterion is highly controlled or compulsive use. The U.S. Surgeon General's report states that "Highly-controlled or compulsive use indicates that drug-seeking and drug-taking behavior is driven by strong, often irresistible urges" (p. 7).

As Warburton (1989) points out, this degree of "compulsion" hardly seems to apply to nicotine. Many smokers have patterns of smoking behavior by which they smoke at work, but not at home, and vice versa. Many refrain from smoking for relatively long periods, for practical or religious reasons, without apparently experiencing any hardship, for example, coal miners who cannot smoke at the pit face and Orthodox Jews who do not smoke on the Sabbath. As Ashton and Stepney (1982) state about these smokers, "The rationale for labelling them as addicts is not convincing" (p. 133). In a similar way, Warburton (1989) examines secondary criteria cited by the U.S. Surgeon General, that is, stereotypic patterns of use, recurrent drug cravings, relapse following abstinence, and induced death by its harmful effects. There is also a set of tertiary criteria, namely that of pleasant or euphoric effect, tolerance, and physical dependence. None of these secondary or tertiary criteria emerge with credit from Warburton's critique, but in view of the widespread belief that physical dependence uniquely defines addiction, it may be worthwhile to consider his critique. As he points out, the existence of physical dependence is an inference made from the abstinence syndrome that occurs when a chronically administered drug is discontinued. Certainly, marked stereotyped symptoms occur after giving up heroin or alcohol. The reported changes after smoking abstinence, however, differ widely from one individual to another and are not present at all in 25% of people giving up smoking. As the APA Diagnostic and Statistical Manual 3-III (1980) observes, discussing nicotine: "In any given case, it is difficult to distinguish a withdrawal effect from the emergence of psychological traits that were suppressed, controlled or altered by the effects of nicotine or from a behavioral reaction (e.g., frustration) to the loss of the reinforcer" (p. 150).

The "Resource" Theory of Smoking

One may conclude from Warburton's (1989) discussion that the term *addiction* is difficult or impossible to define and certainly has no agreed on scientific meaning. The criteria used by the Surgeon General are rather arbitrary, at times trivial, and certainly fail to nail down cigarette smoking as an addiction in any meaningful sense. How then do we explain its prevalence and the difficulties many people have in giving it up?

An alternative way of looking at the situation was suggested by Eysenck (1973). The suggestion is that different people smoke for a variety of reasons, depending on needs in relation to personality, so that they are not *addicted* in any meaningful sense but continue to smoke because they derive certain benefits from smoking, just as they do from eating, drinking, and many other activities. This possibility was first raised by Eysenck, Tarrant, and Woolf (1960) in an article suggesting that perhaps extraverted people smoked because they were bored and wanted to raise their cortical level of arousal, while neurotic people smoked to reduce their tensions and anxieties. While apparently contradictory, both these results can be achieved by varying the amoung of nicotine taken into the bloodstream, nicotine effects apparently being biphasic (Eysenck, 1980). This theory was developed and strengthened by various empirical investigations in later publications (Eysenck, 1973, 1980; Eysenck & O'Connor, 1979).

A typical test of the hypothesis that smoking correlates with extraversion and with associated personality traits diagnostic of sensation seeking has been reported by Knorring and Oreland (1985). In a study of an unselected series of 1,129 eighteen-year-old men from the general Swedish population, they found that regular smokers were extraverted, sensation seeking, easily bored, and with a strong tendency to avoid monotony. These men also had a low level of platelet monoamine oxidase, known to be related to sensation seeking, impulsivity, and extraversion. Ex-smokers had personality traits and platelet monoamine oxidase of the same magnitude as nonsmokers, another indication that smokers and ex-smokers differ in many more ways than just giving up or not giving up smoking.

A study by Frith (1971), analyzing occasions when people smoked cigarettes, provided important evidence to show that, indeed, smokers fell into two clearly marked groups, one class of situations characterized as boring and producing a need to raise cortical arousal, the other characterized by stress of one kind or another, suggesting a need for relaxation. There is now a very large literature on this and related theories, reviewed in detail by Spielberger (1986), and it would not be appropriate to review it again here. By and large, other authors have replicated the original studies but have suggested additional reasons for smoking. Particularly important has been the Tomkins (1968) Affect Control Model, which distinguishes four general types of smoking behavior: (a) positive affect smoking, (b) negative affect smoking, (c) additive smoking, and (d) habitual smoking.

In negative-affect or sedative smoking, according to the theory (Tomkins, 1968), an individual smokes to reduce unpleasant feelings of distress, anger, fear, shame, contempt, or any combination of these primary affects. In contrast, positive-affect smokers generally smoke when they feel good and many never smoke while experiencing negative affect. The addictive-type smokers, according to Tomkins, smoke both to stimulate positive affect and to reduce negative affect. For the habitual smoker, on the other hand, smoking has become an automatic habit, and although habitual smokers may originally have smoked to enhance positive affect, reduce negative affect, or both, affect is no longer associated with smoking.

There are other possible causes, such as increasing attention, and reducing drowsiness, and so on, but it is not the purpose of this chapter to give an extensive list of possible causes for smoking and the needs reduced by smoking. It is sufficient to make the point that smoking does satisfy certain needs of different individuals, depending on their personality, circumstances, and so on.

It should be noted that this discussion concerns the *maintenance* of the smoking habit, which has been shown to be fairly closely related to these needs and to have a strong genetic element (Eysenck, 1980). The origins of the smoking habit relate more to peer pressure, have no strong genetic component, and are not necessarily related to the needs that cause the habit to be maintained, once the habit has been acquired.

Eliminating the Smoking Habit

The value of such an analysis can best be demonstrated by reference to efforts to eliminate the smoking habit. As is well known, traditional methods usually have some effect while the therapy is going on, but once that is finished, the habit is quickly reacquired by most of those who have participated in the therapy. This seems likely to be due to the fact that individual needs still exist, leading to a resumption of smoking, and that the original therapy, being designed for all participants, neglects the individual needs of members of that group.

An effort was made to use the concepts outlined here in improving methods of therapy for smokers by O'Connor and Stravynski (1982). The aim of the study was to validate a situational smoking typology by testing its efficacy in designing reduction strategies. Volunteer smokers were scored on a situational smoking questionnaire that allowed smokers to be classified into high- and low-activity groups on the basis of main cravings. High-activity smokers were further classified into those who smoked either under emotional stress or to aid concentration, whereas low-activity smokers were subdivided into those who smoked to relieve boredom or to relax. From this situational model of motivation, alternative behavioral strategies tailored to the smoker's specific situational demands were devised, in the hope that these might achieve the same effect as smoking and so aid reduction. Thus, smokers who wanted to relieve boredom were taught other methods of doing so, such as playing games, and so on. Patients who were in a high state of anxiety or tenseness were taught methods of relaxation to reduce the anxiety without involving nicotine.

Smokers were allocated at random to one of three treatment groups (O'Connor & Stravynski, 1982). The first was a behavioral substitution group, treated according to the principles outlined here by providing

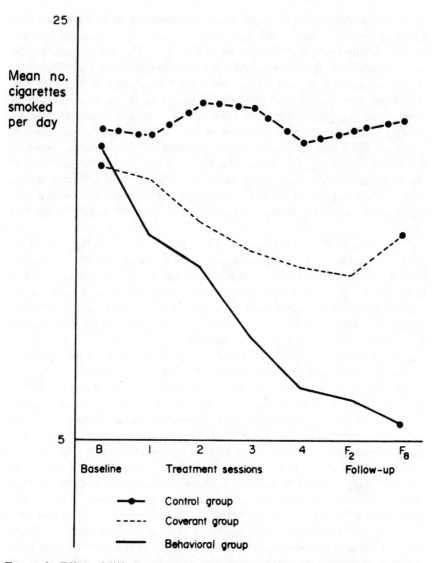

FIGURE 2. Effect of different types of treatment on giving up smoking. (*Note*. From "Evaluation of a Smoking Typology by Use of a Specific Behavioural Substitution Method of Self-Control" by K. O'Connor and A. Stravynski, 1982, *Behaviour Research and Therapy*, *20*, p. 283. Copyright 1982 by Pergamon Press PLC. Reprinted by permission of the publisher and author.)

substitute behavior to replace cigarette smoking. The second group received a generalized coverant approach that emphasized generalized beliefs about smoking effects rather than situational ones; this was a routine procedure in the drug addiction unit at the hospital where the research was done. Finally, there was a no-treatment control group, where subjects only self-monitored their smoking over the treatment period. Results of the treatment are shown in Figure 2. The ordinate shows the mean number of cigarettes smoked per day, the abscissa, the progress of the experiment from a baseline over four treatment sessions to two follow-up sessions, 2 and 8 months respectively, after cessation of treatment. The results are quite clear-cut. The control group showed no change. The behavioral group is about twice as successful as the coverant group in eliminating the habit. Most important of all, however, is a final follow-up that shows a return to the habit on the part of the members of the coverant group, but a continuation of the quitting behavior on the part of the members of the behavioral group. Differences are statistically signifcant between the groups and indicate the value of the need-reduction model.

These results show fairly clearly that the addictive model is inappropriate for most, if not, all smokers. People smoke cigarettes because smoking behavior reduces certain needs and is thus rewarding. When these needs can be met through alternative behaviors, smoking behavior rapidly drops and is eliminated. The addiction model is not suitable for cigarette smoking, and a continued use of the word *addiction* in relation to smoking behavior has no scientific validity.

It is, of course, possible to *define* addictive behavior in psychological terms. Thus, Gossop (1989) defines addiction in functional terms: It is compulsive behavior, that is, under the control of powerful and immediate positive or negative reinforcers, which, when blocked, can produce great distress. Response-prevention elicits powerful unconditioned and conditioned responses. Addiction is characterized by impaired control, that is, correspondence between what addicts say—to themselves or others—and what they do is poor. Finally, addiction persists in the face of evidence or suggestion of harm; long-term consequences of negative valence can be described by addicts, but these consequences exert little control over their behavior. Such a definition is psychologically acceptable, but it clearly generalizes the term *addiction* well beyond the field of drugs; thus, Gossop (1989) deals with sexual crime, gambling, and eating compulsions as addictions. This use might apply to smoking, but it removes the pejorative classification with heroin, LSD, and other addictive drugs.

6
Personality and Stress as Risk Factors

Historically, there has been a great deal of speculation about the possible role of personality and stress as risk factors in the causation of cancer and coronary heart disease (CHD). For cancer, good summaries are found in the works of Bammer and Newberry (1981), Cooper (1983), Hager (1986), Levy (1985), and Pohler (1989). For CHD, the writings of Price (1982) and Steptoe (1981) and relevant and, for stress research in general, a book edited by Cooper (1983). Based on research of this kind, there had been a good deal of interest in the possibility of preventing cancer and CHD by suitable intervention through psychotherapy (Eylenbosch, Depoorter, & Larebeke, 1988).

There has also been much interest in the possibilty of prolonging life through instilling a "fighting spirit" type of reaction in sufferers from cancer and quite generally in the importance of mental attitudes to survival. The evidence certainly suggests that mental attitudes constitute an important prognostic factor in cancer (Eysenck, 1988a; Grossarth-Maticek, 1980a; Greer, Morris, & Pettingale, 1979; Nelson, Friedman, Baer, Lane, & Smith, 1989; Pettingale, Morris, Greer, & Haybittle, 1985; Pettingale, Philalithis, Tee, & Greer, 1981).

Ideas concerning the importance of personality and stress have in recent years been incorporated in a number of theories leading to highly focused investigations. The possibility that type A behavior might be related to and predictive of CHD has received a good deal of attention (Rosenman & Chesney, 1980), but reviews such as those by H.S. Friedman and Booth-Kewley (1987) have suggested that only certain traits of the type A personality, such as anger and aggression, might be related to CHD (Eysenck, 1990b). My work with Grossarth-Maticek and Vetter (Grossarth-Maticek, Eysenck, & Vetter, 1988) certainly supports this view.

A good deal of evidence confirms the relevance of stress to CHD (e.g., Hanson, 1987; Kaplan et al., 1978). Brindley and Rolland (1989) have recently reviewed the evidence, concluding:

An increased control of metabolism by the "stress" or counter-regulatory hormones. . . . is a common feature of [CHD] risk factors. Particular emphasis was placed upon the action of the glucocorticoids—[which] can decrease energy expenditure and, together with insulin, promote energy deposition. These observations provide a partial explanation for the metabolic changes that can accompany the risk factors and clarify why they interact in promoting atherosclerosis. (p. 459)

The Disease-Prone Personality

The cancer-prone personality has often been described as appeasing, unassertive, overcooperative, overpatient, harmony seeking and conflict avoiding, and compliant and defensive (Baltrusch, Stangel, & Waltz, 1988). The two most frequently noted characteristics are (a) suppression of emotional expression and denial of strong emotional reaction and (b) failure to cope successfully with stress and the reaction of giving up, linked with feelings of hopelessness and helplessness (Baltrusch, Stangel, & Waltz, 1988; Eysenck, 1985). This type has sometimes been called "type C," to distinguish it from the CHD-prone type A and the healthy type B (Temoshok, 1987).

Many studies have supported the notion of a "cancer-prone" type, but most of these have been studies comparing individuals suffering from cancer with controls of one kind or another (Eysenck, 1985). Three major prospective studies were mounted to overcome the possibility that the cancer might have caused differences in personality, rather than that personality and stress were risk factors for cancer. There are, of course, several studies along similiar lines. Fox (1978, 1981a, 1981b, 1983, 1988) has critically examined those studies and concluded that results are confusing and contradictory, particularly when the Minnesota Multiple Personality Inventory (Friedman, Webb & Lewak, 1989) was employed as an instrument of personality assessment. It should be noted, however, that most of these studies were heuristic rather than theory based; the use of irrelevant measuring instruments, like the MMPI, cannot invalidate theory-oriented research using appropriate techniques to test these theories. Schmale and Iker (1971) report a study using theoretical concepts similar to those above and find very positive results using an appropriate interviewing procedure; when they used the MMPI as an additional measuring instrument, they obtained entirely negative results. Meta-analyses are quite inappropriate in this field, as in many others (Eysenck, 1984) and should never be used to discount positive outcomes from theory-oriented research. Only failure of replication, appropriately carried out, can be so used.

I (Eysenck, 1990a) have pointed out previously that our results are not unique when proper theory-based and otherwise appropriate measures are used. Meehl (1990), in a very thoughtful monograph entitled "Why Summaries of Research on Psychological Theories Are Often Uninterpretable," has argued for what he calls "a radical and disturbing methodological thesis," which runs as follows: "Null hypothesis testing of correlational predictions from weak substantive theories in soft psychology is subject to the influence of ten obfuscating factors whose effects are usually (1) sizeable, (2) opposed, (3) variable, and (4) unknown. The net epistemic effect of these ten obfuscating factors is that the usual research literature review is well-nigh uninterpretable" (p. 197). Existing reviews of studies linking disease, stress, and personality should be read with this warning in mind.

Three studies have been described in detail by Grossarth-Maticek, Eysenck and Vetter (1988), and only the major results are discussed here. The first of these studies was conducted in a small rural town in Yugoslavia, where every second household was studied, and the oldest inhabitant was used as proband. (There was also an additional small sample of highly stressed people, and occasionally, when the oldest inhabitant was a woman, Yugoslav "macho" attitudes made it necessary to take the oldest man into the sample. These deviations from the research plan had the effect of worsening the outcome, rather than improving it, but the following data are for the total sample.)

The two other studies were conducted in Heidelberg, Germany, and used in the first instance a normal, fairly random sample, with certain age and sex limitations imposed. The second Heidelberg sample was a stressed sample; its members were nominated by members of the normal Heidelberg sample as being under high stress; they were largely friends and relatives of members of the first sample.

Members of these samples were interviewed and given a personality–stress questionnaire; they also gave information concerning their smoking and drinking habits. Blood pressure and blood cholesterol were investigated to provide medical information relevant to these possible risk factors. Mortality was assessed 10 years later.

The personality–stress interviews and questionnaires were used to assign each proband to one of four types. Type 1 was believed to be cancer prone, showing the characteristics outlined here. Type 2 was believed to be CHD prone, again showing a set of characteristics quite different from those of the cancer-prone type. Type 1, in brief, is characterized by understimulation; persons of this type show a permanent tendency to regard an emotionally highly valued object, person, occupation, or whatever as the most important condition for their well-being and happiness. The stress produced by the continued withdrawal or absence of this object is experienced as an emotionally traumatic event. Type-1 individuals fail to distance themselves from the object and remain dependent on it. Thus, individuals of this type do not achieve success in reaching the object and remain distant and isolated from this highly valued and emotionally important object. Great stress is produced by the failure to achieve nearness to the object.

Persons of type 2 (CHD prone) rather show overarousal; they show a continued tendency to regard an emotionally highly important object as the most important cause for their particular distress and unhappiness. Rejection by the object (if a person) or failure to reach it (as in the case of occupational success) is experienced as an emotional trauma, but persons of this type fail to achieve disengagement from the object; rather, they feel more and more helplessly dependent on the object. Thus persons of this type remain in constant contact with these negatively valued and emotionally disturbing people and situations, and fail to distance themselves and free themselves from dependence on the disturbing object, reacting with anger (open or suppressed) and aggression.

The third type, type 3, is characterized by ambivalence. This type shows a tendency to shift from the typical reaction of type 1 to the typical reaction of type 2, and back again. Members show a permanent tendency to regard a highly valued object alternately as the most important condition for his own well-being and as the main cause for their own unhappiness. Individuals of this type experience an alternation of feelings of hopelessness–helplessness and of anger–aggression. Possibly because of this alternation of quite different reaction types, this particular type of proband seems to be relatively safe from both cancer and CHD.

Persons of type 4 are characterized by personal autonomy and in some ways resemble type B of the Friedman-Rosenman typology or the "hardy" personality of Allred and Smith (1989). Persons of this type have a strong tendency to regard their own autonomy, and the autonomy of the persons with whom they wish to be in contact, as the most important condition for their own well-being and happiness. This enables them to experience realistically the approach or avoidance behavior of the object of their desires and thus enables them to accept the autonomy of the object. An inventory to determine which type a proband belongs to has been reproduced by Grossarth-Maticek, Eysenck and Vetter (1988).

Predictions and Mortality

Table 5 shows deaths, and causes of deaths, from various diseases by type of personality in the Yugoslav sample. The crucial figures are the percentage of deaths from cancer in type 1 (46.2%) and the percentage of deaths from CHD in type 2 (29.2%). The figures for both are obviously much lower for types 3 and 4, and the data give substance to the view that personality and stress can be used to predict deaths from cancer and CHD. It will also be clear that type 3 has a high proportion of deaths from other causes, whereas type 4 has the largest percentage of probands still alive.

Table 6 shows deaths from various diseases by types of personality in the Heidelberg normal sample. Here, the number of deaths is much smaller, because the sample is younger than was true of the Yugoslav sample (the

TABLE 5. Causes of death for different types of probands—Yugoslav sample (Grossarth-Maticek, Eysenck, & Vetter, 1988)

Yugoslavia	Living	Cancer	Coronary heart disease	Other causes of deaths	Total
Type 1	72 = 23.8%	140 = 46.2%	25 = 8.3%	66 = 21.8%	303
Type 2	96 = 28.3%	19 = 5.6%	99 = 29.2%	125 = 36.9%	339
Type 3	123 = 56.7%	4 = 1.8%	20 = 9.2%	70 = 32.3%	217
Type 4	437 = 90.7%	3 = .6%	8 = 1.7%	34 = 7.1%	482
Impossible to allocate to type	6	0	4	2	12
Total	734 = 54.2%	166 = 12.3%	156 = 11.5%	297 = 27.0%	1353

Note. Data from "Personality Type, Smoking Habit and Their Interaction as Predictors of Cancer and Coronary Heart Disease" by R. Grossarth-Maticek, H.J. Eysenck, and H. Vetter, 1988, Personality and Individual Differences, 9, p. 486.
Copyright 1989 by Pergamon Press PLC.
Reprinted by permission.

TABLE 6. Causes of death for different types of probands—Heidelberg normal sample (Grossarth-Maticek & Eysenck, 1988)

Heidelberg normal	Living	Cancer	Coronary heart disease	Other causes of deaths	Total
Type 1	78 = 71.6%	19 = 17.4%	2 = 1.8%	10 = 9.2%	109
Type 2	109 = 64.1%	10 = 5.9%	23 = 13.5%	28 = 16.5%	170
Type 3	185 = 98.4%	0	1 = .5%	2 = 1.1%	188
Type 4	387 = 99.0%	0	1 = .3%	3 = .8%	391
Impossible to allocate to type	14	0	0	0	14
Total	773 = 88.6%	29 = 3.3%	27 = 3.1%	43 = 4.9%	872

Note. Data from "Personality Type, Smoking Habit and Their Interaction as Predictors of Cancer and Coronary Heart Disease" by R. Grossarth-Maticek, H.J. Eysenck, and H. Vetter, 1988, Personality and Individual Differences, 9, p. 486.
Copyright 1989 by Pergamon Press PLC.
Reprinted by permission.

average age of the Yugoslav sample was 62 years, that of the Heidelberg normal and Heidelberg stressed sample was 50 years of age.) Clearly, cancer and CHD are diseases of old age, and the 10-year difference in age makes a considerable difference in the number of deaths expected. Nevertheless, the data clearly show again a relationship between cancer and type 1, and CHD and type 2.

TABLE 7. Causes of death for different types of probands—Heidelberg stressed sample

Heidelberg stressed group	Living	Cancer	Coronary heart disease	Other causes of deaths	Total (n)
Type 1	188 = 38.4%	188 = 38.4%	34 = 7.0%	79 = 16.2%	489
Type 2	148 = 47.9%	7 = 2.3%	86 = 27.8%	68 = 22.0%	309
Type 3	153 = 92.7%	4 = 2.4%	0	8 = 4.8%	165
Type 4	71 = 97.3%	0	0	2 = 2.7%	73
Impossible to allocate to type	6	0	0	0	6
Total	556 = 54.3%	199 = 19.1%	120 = 11.5%	157 = 15.1%	1042

Note. Data from "Personality Type, Smoking Habit and Their Interaction as Predictors of Cancer and Coronary Heart Disease" by R. Grossarth-Maticek, H.J. Eysenck, and H. Vetter, 1988, *Personality and Individual Differences, 9*, p. 487. Copyright 1989 by Pergamon Press PLC. Reprinted by permission.

Table 7 shows deaths from various diseases by type of personality in the Heidelberg stressed sample. Here, the number of the deaths is much closer to that in the Yugoslav study, in spite of the difference of 10 years of age; because the two Heidelberg samples are very similar in all other respects, it seems reasonable to attribute this larger number of deaths to the stress experienced by this group. In the Heidelberg normal sample, 88.6% were still alive at the end of this 10-year follow-up; in the Heidelberg stressed sample, only 54.3% were still alive. This difference is suggestive of the importance of stress in causing death.

The data can be inspected more directly in the form of Figures 3 to 5, which show clearly how close is the relation between personality type and disease.

When first published, these results appeared almost too good to be true and a further $4\frac{1}{2}$-year follow-up was planned under an independent group of international experts who closely supervised this extension of the two Heidelberg studies. The results have now come in, but have not yet been published. The trends observed during the first 10 years continued without change, suggesting that the relationship between personality–stress and disease is truly as close as suggested in these data. Figure 6 gives the results for the two Heidelberg samples combined.

Several explicit or implicit replications of these studies show similar relationships. I have reviewed earlier studies elsewhere (Eysenck, 1985). More recent studies are those of Kune, Kune, Watson, and Bahnson (in press); Quander-Blaznik (1991); Beek; Schmitz, 1990; and Wirsching, Stierlin, Weber, Wirsching, and Hoffman (1981). Of particular interest is the work of Baalen and de Vries (1987), who showed that in patients with

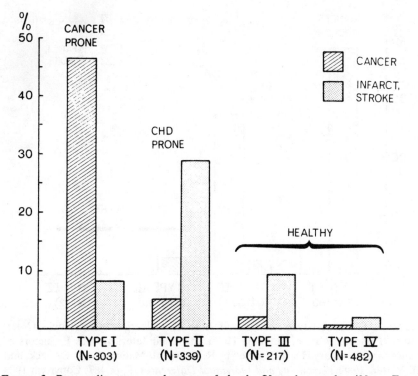

FIGURE 3. Personality type and cause of death, Yugoslav study. (*Note.* From "Personality Type, Smoking Habit and Their Interaction as Predictors of Cancer and Coronary Heart Disease" by R. Grossarth-Maticek, M.J. Eysenck, and H. Vetter, 1988, *Personality and Individual Differences*, 9, p. 486. Copyright 1988 by Pergamon Press PLC. Reprinted by permission.)

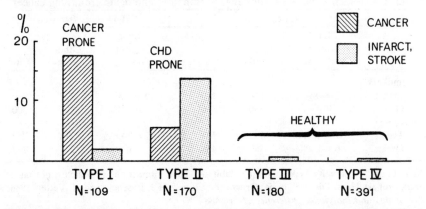

FIGURE 4. Personality type and cause of death, Heidelberg normal sample. (*Note.* From "Personality Type, Smoking Habit and Their Interaction as Predictors of Cancer and Coronary Heart Disease" by R. Grossarth-Maticek, M.J. Eysenck, and H. Vetter, 1988, *Personality and Individual Differences*, 9, p. 487. Copyright 1988 by Pergamon Press PLC. Reprinted by permission.)

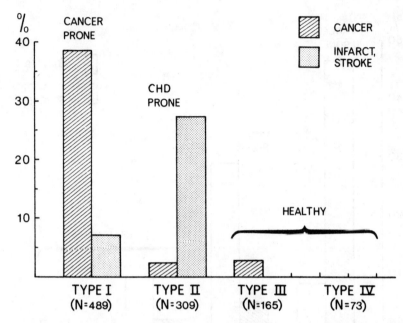

FIGURE 5. Personality type and cause of death, Heidelberg stressed sample. (*Note.*
From "Personality Type, Smoking Habit and Their Interaction as Predictors of
Cancer and Coronary Heart Disease" by R. Grossarth-Maticek, M.J. Eysenck, and
H. Vetter, 1988, *Personality and Individual Differences*, *9*, p. 487. Copyright 1988
by Pergamon Press PLC. Reprinted by permission.)

TABLE 8. Interaction between smoking, personality, and death from lung cancer

	Yugoslavia			Heidelberg (stressed)		
	Lung cancer deaths	Other deaths	Total	Lung cancer deaths	Other deaths	Total
Nonsmokers						
Type 1	1 = .8%	118	119	9 = 3.8%	227	236
Others	0	550	550	3 = 1.0%	297	300
Smokers						
Type 1	31 = 16.9%	153	184	37 = 14.6%	216	253
Others	6 = 1.2%	482	488	0	247	247

Note. From "Personality Type, Smoking Habit and Their interaction as Predictors of Cancer
and Coronary Heart Disease" by R. Grossarth-Maticek, H.J. Eysenck, and H. Vetter, 1988,
Personality and Individual Differences, *9*, p. 488.
Copyright 1988 by Pergamon Press.
Reprinted by permission.

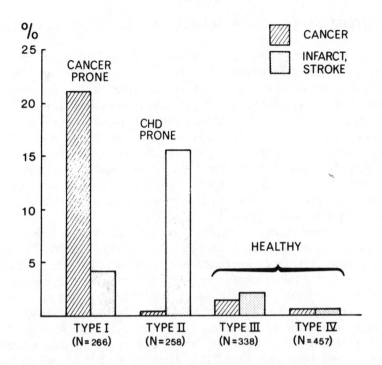

FIGURE 6. Personality and cause of death, Heidelberg combined samples, 1982 to 1986. Unpublished study, Grossarth-Maticek and Eysenck.

extensive metastases who recovered without operations or chemotherapy, all had personalities resembling those of type 4.

The importance of smoking for the type–cancer relationship must now be considered. Table 8 shows the number of cancer deaths, other deaths, and total deaths for nonsmokers and smokers of type 1, as compared with individuals of the other three types. Among nonsmokers, as expected, there are very few deaths from lung cancer, but of the 13 that occurred, 10 occurred in persons of type 1. For smokers, there were 74 deaths, only 6 of which occurred in persons other than type 1. These results give rise to an association between type 1 and lung cancer of $p = .0001$ for both the samples considered when a correction has been made for differences in smoking habits according to the Mantel-Haenszel (1959) formula. It is clear that quite independent of smoking, individuals of type 1 are cancer prone, as compared with individuals of types 2, 3, and 4. (See also Grossarth-Maticek, Eysenck, & Vetter, 1988.)

Synergistic Interaction Between Smoking and Personality

Table 8 (Grossarth-Maticek, Eysenck, & Vetter, 1988) makes clear that there is a synergistic interaction between smoking and typology. The only group that has a high proportion of deaths from lung cancer is that of smokers of type 1; smokers not of type 1, and nonsmokers either of type 1 or of the other types have negligible rates of cancer deaths. Of the two factors, smoking and personality, personality seems to be the stronger. Of 735 smokers not of type 1, only 6 were found to have died of lung cancer; this number is not very different from 3 nonsmokers not of type 1 who died out of the 850 individuals who were nonsmokers. Clearly, smoking appears to represent a danger to health as far as lung cancer is concerned mainly for individuals of type 1.

The data may deserve a slightly more formal analysis, following the traditional methods of epidemiology (D.A. Perkins, 1989). The background factor for the two populations (Yugoslav & Heidelberg stressed; Eysenck, 1988b) taken together is 0.35% for lung cancer mortality ($N = 850$). For personality in nonsmokers, it is 2.89%, giving an excess of 2.54% (2.89% − 0.35%), which may be called the *stress effect*. For smoking in personality other than type 1, the effect is 0.45% (0.80% − 0.35%), that is, about a fifth of that of stress. The combined effect of smoking and personality is 15.21% (15.56% − 0.35%), which is five times the effect expected from simple addition of the smoking and personality effects (0.45% + 2.54% = 2.99%). Thus, synergism produces a 500% increase in cancer mortality from smoking and personality, highly significant using a log linear contingency table modeling formula.

This calculation is made for 2,374 people, giving 77 cases of lung cancer mortality; the numbers clearly are not large enough to take the resulting calculations as anything but a very "rough and ready" guideline. Also, it may be objected that the calculation brings together two rather unlike populations (Yugoslav & German), differing in age and stress (Grossarth-Maticek, Eysenck, & Vetter, 1988). Both groups, however, give similar results when analyzed independently and hence may not be too dissimilar for the purpose of analysis. (The Heidelberg normal group had too few cases of lung cancer to be included.)

A replication study was carried out with 1,914 probands. The results for lung cancer were as follows, defining *stress* and *no stress* in terms of belonging or not belonging to type 1. The percentage of lung cancer mortality was .69% for no-stress nonsmokers, 2.09% for stressed nonsmokers, .24% for no-stress smokers, but 10.59% for stressed smokers. This gives an additive effect of stress plus smoking of .95%, but an actual effect of 10.59% − .69% = 9.90%, making the synergistic effect equal to 8.95%. This, again, is highly significant statistically.

On the same population we looked at CHD, using belonging to Type 2 behavior as the criterion of stress. The background factor here was 1.10%

mortality from CHD for nonstress nonsmokers, 5.30% for stressed nonsmokers, 3.04% for nonstress smokers, but 17.50% for stressed smokers. This gives an additive effect for stress and smoking of 6.14% + 1.10% = 7.14%, but an actual effect of 17.50%, making the synergistic effect equal to 10.36%. In both cases, the stress effect is significantly greater than the smoking effect, but what is truly outstanding is the synergistic effect.

While these data are of a kind to show even by visual inspection that there is a strong interaction, and while analysis using an *additive* model clearly suggests such a view, this is not the only available model (Cox, 1970; Darrock, 1974; Galtung, 1967, p. 415; Grizzle et al., 1969; and Plackett, 1974). There is also a *multiplicative*, logistic model (Everitt, 1977), and the two models may give quite different answers, as Everitt and Smith (1979) point out in discussing alternative interpretations of identical data by Brown and Harris (1978) and Tennant and Bebbington (1978). Briefly, the essential difference between the two models is that the additive one looks simply at *differences between proportions*, while the multiplicative models work with *ratios* of proportions, or relative risks. As Everitt and Smith (1979) point out, "it is quite possible for the 2 models to lead to seemingly conflicting results when applied to the same set of data." (p. 582). In the case of the above Table, the logistic analysis gives a result in terms of *independent* variables *not* interacting with each other.

Which model is the correct one? As Everitt and Smith point out, "unfortunately there is no absolute answer, and in practice the choice between them may depend on rather complex reasoning." (p. 582). Linear rather than logistic analysis using a log-linear model, is perhaps more direct, and gives us a clear answer to a most practical question: which of the four groups in our table is the one we should direct our effort toward when suggesting giving up smoking and learning, too, to cope with stress? I have proceeded in the discussion on the basis of the linear, additive model, but readers should be warned that there exists an alternative model which may have to be considered in future discussions of this problem. (Other alternatives are the probit and the complementary log-log functions).

It would take us too far out of the discussion to consider in detail the reasons for choosing an additive rather than a multiplicative model; the references given suggest that for data such as those of Brown and Harris (1978), or those here considered, which posit two separate and largely independent risk factors against a known background of risk enable us to postulate a natural scale upon which to search for interaction in effects where the factors can be conceptualized as, say, physical (smoking) or psychological (stress) insults to the organism. The interaction term would then suggest that the effects of our "insult" would be stronger in an organism already subjected to another "insult." The available data do not prove this analysis to be correct; they merely render it likely.

Ultimately, of course, there is no real inconsistency between outcomes. As the names imply, the additive model adds separate effects, and finds a huge interaction effect; the multiplicative model multiplies separate effects (on a different scale) and fails to find interaction effects because these have been incorporated into the process of multiplying effects. The main point remains that effects are synergistic, with interaction in additive models, or with multiplicative effects in multiplicative models.

We (Grossarth-Maticek, Eysenck, & Vetter, 1988) have carried out similar analyses for other risk factors (blood pressure, blood cholesterol) and compared these with smoking as a risk factor. We performed these analyses for all three samples, that is, the Yugoslav, the Heidelberg normal, and the Heidelberg stressed sample. The results are quite similar, no matter which dependent variable, organic variable or place of investigation is considered. Table 9 shows the results.

1. The organic variable has different relevance for mortality, depending on the psychosocial type. Its relevance is greatest with that type that itself has the greatest specific mortality, that is, type 1 for cancer and type 2 for CHD. The psychosocial types are relevant, not only for mortality, but in a similar way for sensitivity to organic risk factors.

2. The psychosocial types do show differences with respect to the organic variables, but these differences cannot explain away the relevance of the types for mortality; according to the figures for mortality, type-specific mortality differences when adjusted for differences of the organic variables are still highly significant.

These data suggest several conclusions. Psychosocial variables, and particularly personality type and stress, are important in mediating deaths from cancer and CHD. These personality variables are more influential than physical factors like smoking, blood pressure, and cholesterol, in the ratio of roughly 6:1 for the groups here studied.

Finally, personality and physical factors interact synergistically. These are important findings for any attempt to prevent deaths from cancer and CHD.

The findings that risk factors in cancer and CHD act synergistically, not by simple addition, is so important that these findings may be amplified by two studies (Grossarth-Maticek & Eysenck, in press-a.) One of these is summarized in Table 10.

Table 10 shows the results of a study comparing death rates of probands having 1, and 2, and 3, or all 4 of four different risk factors. The risk factors were (a) smoking (more than 20 cigarettes per day for over 10 years); (b) heredity (at least one first-degree relative suffering from or died of lung cancer); (c) chronic bronchitis; and (d) stress, that is, probands of type 1 or 2. Not all combinations of risk factors could be found in sufficient numbers, but the data show very clearly the synergistic effects of multiplying risks.

As shown in Table 10, among these probands at 13-year follow-up (average age between 51 and 54 years old at the beginning of the study),

TABLE 9. Relative importance of personality and organic risk factors for death

		Mean			b			Mort. (%)	
Type	Y	H1	H2	Y	H1	H2	Y	H1	H2
rf: systolic blood pressure									
dis.: infarct/stroke mortality									
1	151.0	—	174.2	.056	—	.024	7.6	—	7.2
2	160.7	—	207.6	.084	—	.108	27.2	—	23.7
3	148.3	—	186.3	.005	—	.010	7.7	—	2.3
4	144.6	—	185.8	.003	—	.021	1.8	—	5.0
all	150.7	—	187.7	.035	—	.041	11.1	—	9.1
Significance of differences	.0000		.0000	.0004		.0011	<.0001		<.0001
rf: diastolic blood pressure									
dis.: infarct/stroke mortality									
1	90.0	—	85.8	.026	—	.019	5.1	—	7.2
2	93.7	—	93.5	.093	—	.071	26.8	—	24.5
3	88.6	—	88.9	.020	—	.004	8.5	—	2.5
4	86.8	—	89.0	.014	—	.007	2.1	—	5.5
all	89.6	—	88.8	.038	—	.025	10.6	—	9.9
Significance of differences	.0000		.0000	.0137		.0494	<.0001		<.0001
rf: blood cholesterol									
dis.: infarct/stroke mortality									
1	255.6	217.5	258.3	.011	.004	.037	8.3	3.2	8.5
2	250.4	254.4	305.1	.036	.054	.046	29.4	9.7	24.7
3	245.8	216.8	282.6	.027	.000	.003	9.2	1.8	1.8
4	245.5	217.9	280.5	.001	.001	.000	1.8	.8	3.5
all	249.1	224.9	277.8	.019	.014	.020	12.2	3.9	9.6
Significance of differences	.0330	.0000	.0000	NS	NS	.0486	<.0001	.0008	.0000
rf: cigarettes per day									
dis.: infarct/stroke mortality									
1	15.7	13.0	16.9	.00	.003	.000	7.7	4.1	6.9
2	10.4	18.8	14.4	.038	.050	.161	29.8	12.0	27.6
3	11.6	8.9	12.2	.021	.016	.007	8.3	2.5	1.7
4	10.8	8.2	10.9	.002	.008	.011	1.8	1.2	3.5
all	11.9	11.1	15.0	.005	.019	.045	11.9	5.0	9.9

TABLE 9. (Cont.)

Type	Mean			b			Mort. (%)		
	Y	H1	H2	Y	H1	H2	Y	H1	H2
Significance of differences	.0000	.0000	.0000	NS	NS	.0000	<.0001	.0002	.0001
rf: cigarettes per day									
dis.: lung cancer mortality									
1	15.7	13.0	16.9	.075	.019	.044	8.2	3.6	8.3
2	10.4	18.8	14.4	.020	.010	.003	2.5	2.5	1.5
3	11.6	8.9	12.2	.003	.015	.007	1.3	2.4	1.7
4	10.8	8.2	10.9	.002	.008	.011	0.6	1.2	3.5
all	11.9	11.1	15.0	.025	.013	.016	3.1	2.4	3.7
Significance of differences	.0000	.0000	.0000	.0001	NS	.0113	<.0001	NS	.0000

largest (abs.) value is underlined

For Yugoslavia, the organic variables represent a single measurement taken in 1966 (cholesterol: 1969).
For Heidelberg, the organic variables are the average of up to 7 measurements take in 1972.
Abbreviations:

rf = risk factor.

dis. = disease.

mean = mean of organic variable within type groups.

b = regression coefficient of the dependent variable on the organic variable within type groups.

mort. = mortality (the dependent variable) within type groups, adjusted for the organic variable.

Y = Yugoslavia H1 = Heidelberg representative H2 = Heidelberg stressed. NS means $p > .05$.

Note. From "Personality Type, Smoking Habit and Their Interaction as Predictors of Cancer and Coronary Heart Disease" by R. Grossarth-Maticek, H.J. Eysenck, and H. Vetter, 1988, Personality and Individual Differences, 9, p. 489.
Copyright 1988 by Pergamon Press PLC.
Reprinted by permission.

none had died of lung cancer among those who only showed one risk factor. Of those showing two risk factors, only about 1% died of lung cancer. Combinations of three risk factors showed quite elevated death rates for lung cancer, varying from 7.6% through 9.8% to 20%. Combinations of four risk factors raised the death rate from lung cancer to 31%, demonstrating the strong synergistic effect of multiplying risk factors.

Of particular interest in Table 10 is the group of four risk-factor probands in brackets, they had received prophylactic behavior therapy (BT) and, accordingly, had a death rate from lung cancer only about one third as high as the group of four risk-factor probands who received no therapy. Thus, even for those most exposed to lung cancer, prophylactic treatment is possible and can be efficacious. Chapter 7 deals with the prophylactic effects of behavior therapy.

A final study may be mentioned here to indicate the independent effects of smoking and stress (Grossarth-Maticek & Eysenck, in press-a). This study concerned 1,256 men with stress and 1,256 men without stress, equated for age; none suffered from bronchitis or hereditary predisposition (defined in terms of first-degree relatives suffering from or dying of cancer.) The dependent variable is the number of probands in each group dying of lung cancer. Figure 7 shows the results. Clearly, smoking shows a dose-response curve implicating it as a risk factor for lung cancer. Stress similarly acts as a risk factor for lung cancer.

It would not be true to say that smoking and stress constitute the only major risk factors; another is genetic predisposition. This, too, interacts

TABLE 10. Synergistic effects of H (heredity), B (chronic bronchitis), C (cigarette smoking), and S (stress–personality); effects of BT (behavior therapy)

Combination of risks	n	Lung cancer	%	Other causes of death	%	Average age
Only H	50	0	0	5	10	51
Only C	100	0	0	12	12	52
Only S	59	0	0	16	27	52
H + C	50	1	2	4	8	53
H + B	52	0	0	8	15	51
C + B	55	0	0	11	20	52
C + S	100	2	2	21	21	53
H + S	49	0	0	9	18	54
B + S	50	0	0	8	16	53
C + H + B	26	2	8	5	19	51
C + H + S	50	10	20	14	28	51
C + B + S	51	5	10	10	20	51
· H + C + B + S	26	8	31	8	31	52
[H + C + B + S + BT]	26	3	12	4	15	52

Note. Data from "Personality and Stress as Synergistic Risk Factors for Cancer and Coronary Heart Disease, in Interaction with Smoking, Genetic, Predisposition, and Chronic Bronchitis" by R. Grossarth-Maticek and H.J. Eysenck, in press-a, Integrative Physiological and Behavioral Science.

synergistically with stress (Grossarth-Maticek & Eysenck, in press-a). Figure 8 shows the number of probands dying of lung cancer when plotted against the number of first-degree relatives dying of, or suffering from, lung cancer; stressed and nonstressed probands, defined as being or not being of type 1, are plotted separately. There is a clear linear relation between the degree of genetic predisposition and the mortality rate, but equally clearly, stress interacts powerfully with genetic predisposition to produce a synergistic effect.

It is important to be clear about the contribution of heredity. There may be a contribution to cancerogenesis or to the adequacy of the immune

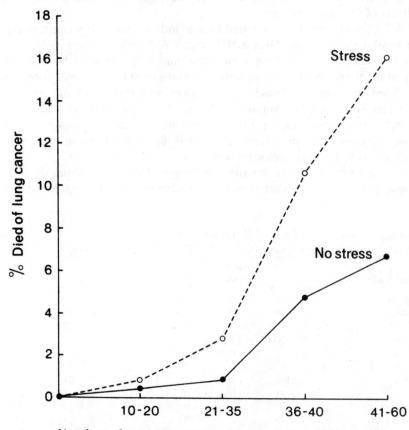

FIGURE 7. Combined action of two risk factors for cancer. (*Note.* From "Personality and Stress as Synergistic Risk Factors for Cancer and Coronary Heart Disease, in Interaction With Smoking, Genetic Predisposition, and Chronic Bronchitis" by R. Grossarth-Maticek and H.J. Eysenck, in press-a, *Integrative Physiological and Behavioral Science.* Copyright 1991, by H.J. Eysenck. Reprinted by permission.)

system. There may be a contribution to the personality factors that determine suppression of the emotions (Eaves, Eysenck, & Martin, 1989). And finally, there may be a contribution to the occurrence of stress itself. It is often assumed that the events listed in such scales as the Holmes and Rahe (1967) Social Readjustment Rating Scale just happen to the person concerned, but this is incorrect; as Plomin and Bergeman (in press) have shown, many of these discontents are self-caused, and "the model fitting estimate of heritability is 40% for the total life event outcome." A more detailed analysis of the genetic contribution to cancer and CHD is long overdue.

It should not be assumed that the notion of *synergistic* action finds support only in the Grossarth-Maticek and Eysenck studies. In a recent paper, D.A. Perkins (1989) has argued that interactions among the major coronary heart disease risk factors of smoking, hypertension, and elevated cholesterol may contribute substantially to the prediction of CHD risks over and above the sum of the independent risks due to their factors (p. 3). He surveys results that show that the interaction of smoking and cholesterol and of hypertension and cholesterol may each as much as

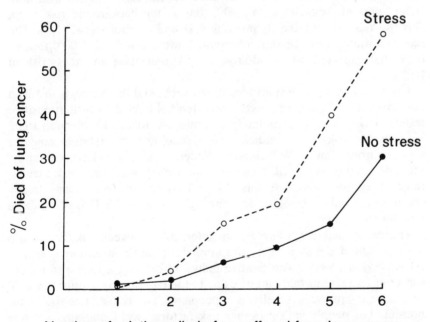

FIGURE 8. Stress and genetic predisposition as risk factors for lung cancer. (*Note.* From "Personality and Stress as Synergistic Risk Factors for Cancer and Coronary Heart Disease, in Interaction With Smoking, Genetic Predisposition, and Chronic Bronchitis" by R. Grossarth-Maticek and H.J. Eysenck, in press-a, *Integrative Physiological and Behavioral Science.* Copyright 1991, by H.J. Eysenck. Reprinted by permission.)

double the risks of CHD which might be expected if these factors acted only additively (p. 3). He also comments on the strong possibilty of an interaction between chronic psychosocial stress and elevated cholesterol (p. 3). Other authors who have argued in favor of synergistic interaction effects are Kleinbaum, Kupper, and Morganstern (1982); Rothman (1974); Rothman and Keller (1972); Kannel, Neaton, & Wentworth (1986); and Saracci (1987), K.A. Perkins (1985, 1987), Walker (1981), and Kooperman (1981) have also added to the methodological analysis of synergistic effects.

An example will illustrate methods and results. Kannel, Neaton, & Wentworth (1986) have reported data on over 300,000 white men selected for inclusion in the Multiple Risk Factor Intervention Trial (MRFIT) mentioned in Chapter 1. For men between 35 and 45 years of age, in the lowest quintile of diastolic blood pressure (<76 mmHg), the 6-year risk of CHD mortality among nonsmokers without elevated cholesterol (i.e., background risks) was .6/1,000, whereas the risk resulting from smoking alone was 1.0/1,000 and the risk for nonsmokers with cholesterol in the highest quintile (>2.44 mg/dL) was 2.0/1,000. If the effects of smoking and elevated cholesterol were only additive, the risk of those with both factors present would be 2.44/1,000, that is, the background risk of .6, plus the risk attributable to smoking (.4) and to cholesterol (1.4). The actual mortality rate for this subgroup, however, was 4.8/1,000, that is, *twice* that expected on an additive model, indicating an excess risk of 100%!

This is clearly an important area of research, and the concepts involved may explain why *single* risk factors so often fail to give consistent positive results. It is certainly completely inadmissible to use simple univariate analyses for risk-factor studies in epidemiology; multivariate analyses are an absolute must (Wilhelmsen, Wedel, & Tibblin, 1973). Certainly, smoking emerges as a risk factor in conjunction with other risk factors, rather than by itself. For this, as well as for other reasons already adumbrated, talk of smoking as "causing" cancer of CHD is of doubtful scientific relevance.

The established facts of synergistic interaction between risk factors also have profound consequences for prophylaxis and prevention generally (D.A. Perkins, 1989). The relative failure of quitting smoking to reduce cancer and CHD mortality may be due to the fact that such quitting would only have any pronounced effects in people with more than one risk factor present. For people with no other risk factors except smoking, quitting smoking would have little effect on mortality, and their inclusion in any study would disguise any impact that quitting smoking might have on mortality.

This certainly is the implication of the published data summarized in this chapter and particularly of Table 9. Quitting smoking in persons of type 4 would only have a minimal effect, if any, on mortality.

(For readers who would like more detailed information on the Grossarth-Maticek personality types, the Appendix lists the questions in a short version of the questionnaire, which has been used in more recent studies [Grossarth-Maticek, & Eysenck, 1990]. In these later studies, two more types have been added to the four types already mentioned, type 5 relating specifically to rheumatoid arthritis, as well as to cancer, and type 6 to drug addiction. Type 5 is characterized by rational-antiemotional behavior, and type 6 by antisocial, psychopathic behavior.)

7
Intervention Studies in Cancer and Coronary Heart Disease

In Chapter 6, I attempted to demonstrate that psychosocial factors such as stress and personality are important risk factors in the causation of cancer and coronary heart disease (CHD) and that specific personality constellations, reacting to stress, are particularly cancer prone and CHD prone. These relationships, although much stronger than those linking smoking to cancer and CHD, are still only correlational, and it is well-known that *correlations cannot be used directly to infer causation*. The best way to indicate that the relations observed are indeed causal is by some intervention method that brings to bear an experimental paradigm on the problem in question. Grossarth-Maticek and I have attempted to do this by using methods of behavior therapy (Eysenck & Martin, 1987) in an attempt to alter the behavior of the cancer-prone or the CHD-prone person in the direction of the healthy type 4. In other words, we have attempted to increase autonomous behavior and reduce the proband's dependence on other people or his acceptance of situations that lead to negative consequences. This section includes a brief discussion of the methods used and then an evaluation of the effects of using these methods for prophylaxis. (For a more general discussion of prophylactic methods, see Aeberhardt, 1989.)

The therapy developed by us contains many familiar features, such as Wolpe's method of desensitization, Lazarus's development of coping mechanisms, social skills training, and others. The method has been called *autonomy training* or *creative novation behavior therapy*. The major aim of the treatment is to stimulate an individual to look toward the long-term positive results of different types of behavior and self-evaluation (Grossarth-Maticek & Eysenck, 1991). Thus, the treatment aims to increase behaviors that lead to long-term positive consequences, even though this may involve some short-term negative consequences. Conversely, the patient should learn to avoid behaviors that lead to long-term negative consequences, even if these may be associated with short-term positive consequences.

Psychological Therapy in Prevention of Cancer and CHD

Having briefly described the methods of prophylactic behavior therapy, the following discussion considers their application to a variety of probands of types 1 and 2, that is people prone to cancer and CHD, respectively. Grossarth-Maticek and I have conducted three major studies, using, respectively, long-term individual therapy, group therapy, and bibliotherapy conjoined with short individual therapy. These studies will be discussed with respect to death, cause of death (as shown on the death certificate), and incidence, that is, the diagnosis of cancer or CHD made by the patient's physician and ascertained with the patients prior permission. All the studies were carried out in Heidelberg (Germany), and the therapist in each case with Professor Grossarth-Maticek, who originated the methods used (Eysenck & Grossarth-Maticek, 1991; Grossarth-Maticek & Eysenck, 1991).

Probands in the first of these studies, using long-term individual therapy, were 100 individuals, 50 men and 50 women, who were categorized as type 1 (cancer prone) on the basis of interview and questionnaire data. Their mean age was around 50 years. The second group of 92 individuals,

TABLE 11. Effects of behavior therapy on 50 cancer-prone and 46 coronary heart disease-prone probands compared with controls, follow-up 1972–1986

I. Cancer	n	Deaths	Diseased	Other causes of death	Living
Control	50	23	—	15	17
Incidence		46%		30%	34%
Therapy	50	2	—	5	44
Incidence		4%		10%	88%
Total	100	25		20	61
Incidence					

II. CHD	n	Deaths	Diseased	Other causes of deaths	Living
Control	46	16	20	13	17
Incidence		34.8%	43.5%	28.3%	36.9%
Therapy	46	3	11	6	37
Incidence		6.5%	23.9%	13%	80.4%
Total	92	19	31	19	54
Incidence		20.6%	33.7%	20.7%	58.7%

Note. Data updated from "Creative Novation Behaviour Therapy as a Prophylactic Treatment for Cancer and Coronary Heart Disease: 2. Effects of Treatment, H.J. Eysenck and R. Grossarth-Maticek 1991. *Behaviour Research and Therapy, 29*, p. 17–31.

similarly selected, but all of type 2, were chosen to study the effects of behavior therapy on CHD. The therapy consisted of roughly 30 hours of individual therapy, as outlined at the beginning of this chapter. The results are shown in Table 11. Both for cancer and for CHD, the number of deaths is very significantly less for the therapy group than for the control group. The same is true for incidence, which is roughly half in the therapy group as compared with the control group. These data suggest very strongly that behavior therapy can prevent death from cancer or CHD, or at least postpone it for a very considerable period of time. It is, of course, possible that the surviving members in the therapy group will ultimately die of cancer or CHD, or at least some of them will; only a much longer follow-up, until all the participants of the study are dead, can answer this question. What is shown is that 13 years after the initiation of the study, many more members of the therapy group are alive than of the control group.

It should also be noted that details of all probands were transmitted to two independent observers before death and cause of death, or incidence, were ascertained in each case. In addition, a random sample of inter-viewers was interviewed by an independent observer to check on the collection of interview and questionnaire data. These precautions were taken as a routine measure to certify the *objectivity* of the data collection.

Our second study is concerned with group behavior therapy. In this case, we formed groups of between 20 and 25 probands, and administered group behavior therapy for periods of between 6 and 25 hours, each group meeting lasting between 2 and 3 hours. Duration was determined by the members of the groups themselves and hence varied to a considerable

TABLE 12. Effects of group behavior therapy on cancer and coronary heart disease, eight-year follow-up

	Therapy (n = 245) (Not contacted = 6)		Control (n = 245) (Not contacted = 11)	
	Mortality	Diseased	Mortality	Diseased
	239	235	234	231
Cancer	18	75	111	129
Incidence	7.5%	31.9%	47.4%	55.8%
Coronary heart disease	10	29	36	45
Incidence	4.2%	12.3%	15.4%	19.5%
Other causes of death	20	—	33	—
Incidence	8.4%		14.1%	
Living	191		56	
Incidence	79.9%		23.9%	

Note. Data from "Creative Novation Behaviour Therapy as a Prophylactic Treatment for Cancer and Coronary Heart Disease: 2. Effects of Treatment H.J. Eysenck and R. Grossarth-Maticek 1991. *Behaviour Research and Therapy, 29,* p. 20.

degree. Matching was carried out as before, and members of the group were followed up over an 8-year period. Results are given in Table 12.

It will be seen that group therapy, very much like long-term individual therapy, benefitted the therapy group, as compared with the control group, by reducing the mortality from cancer and CHD and decreasing the incidence. Given the relative unreliability of diagnoses as recorded on death certificates, the most impressive figure perhaps is that of the proportion still living, which indicates the power of behavior therapy to prevent cancer and CHD. Again, the procedure, including all the death certificates, was checked by an independent observer (Eysenck & Grossarth-Maticek, 1991).

Our third study concerned a special kind of bibliotherapy, which centered on a text entitled "How to Achieve Emotional Independence and a Healthy Personality." This text was introduced to participants in an hour-long introduction by Professor Grossarth-Maticek, who also outlined the application of the principles contained therein to the individual proband. After a week or so—to give the proband time to read and understand the test and to try to apply it to his own condition—specially trained students discussed this application of the message contained in the text to the individual's circumstances, for three 1-hour periods. Therefore, this study concerned not just bibliotherapy but in addition some 4 hours of individual therapy.

In this study, the therapy group consisted of 600 probands, matched as before with a control group of 600. Again, we allocated probands on a chance basis to therapy or control. Within the control group, a small group of 100 was exposed to a placebo treatment, that is, using a psychoanalytic text outlining Freudian ideas concerning the origins and prevention of cancer. Table 13 shows the results of the study. It will be seen that the placebo group does not differ significantly from the control group, but the therapy group is superior to the control group both with respect to smaller number of deaths from cancer and CHD, and lower incidence of these two diseases. The data show that even a relatively short-term application of behavior therapy, together with bibliotherapy, can have a marked effect on mortality and incidence of cancer and CHD (Eysenck & Grossarth-Maticek, 1991).

It is important to note that not all methods of psychological interventions are successful in preventing cancer and CHD, and some may indeed have the opposite effect of increasing the probability of disease. Grossarth-Maticek and I (Grossarth-Maticek & Eysenck, 1990) have shown that psychoanalysis has a very negative effect on health, increasing mortality from cancer and CHD substantially. A kind of dose–response relationship exists here; the longer exposure to psychoanalysis, the greater is the mortality. Short-term psychotherapy was not found to have any positive or negative effects, compared with control groups. These findings contradict the view that simply showing compassion, talking with people, and

TABLE 13. Effects of bibliotherapy and short behavior therapy on cancer and coronary heart disease (CHD) thirteen-year follow-up

| | Causes of Death | | | | | | | | Not investigated | |
| | Cancer | | CHD | | Other | | Total | Living | | |
	M	D	M	D	M	D			M	D
Control (n = 500)	106	162	145	203	164	—	415	78	7	15
Incidence	21.5%	33.4%	29.4%	41.8%	33.3%	—	84.2%	15.8%	1.4%	3%
Control with use of psychoanalytic text (placebo group) (n = 100)	22	37	31	40	28	—	81	19	0	2
Incidence	22%	37.7%	31%	40.8%	28%	—	81%	19%	0%	2%
Therapy group with behavior therapy text (n = 600)	27	99	47	132	115	—	189	409	2	14
Incidence	4.5%	16.9%	7.9%	22.5%	19.2%	—	31.6%	68.4%	.3%	2.3

CHD, coronary heart disease; D, diseased; M, mortality.
Note. Data from "Creative Novation Behaviour Therapy as a Prophylactic Treatment for Cancer and Coronary Heart Disease: 2. Effects of Treatment H.J. Eysenck and R. Grossarth-Maticek 1991. *Behaviour Research and Therapy, 29*, p. 20.

generally interacting with them would have beneficial effects; apparently, it is the *content* of the interventions that is the important part of the treatment.

More detailed information concerning our studies of intervention is given by Eysenck 1988a, 1988b, 1989; Grossarth-Maticek, Bastiaans, and Kanazir, 1985; Grossarth-Maticek, Eysenck, and Vetter, 1988; and Grossarth-Maticek, Schmidt, Vetter, and Arndt, 1984. These communications also contain information on the possibilities of prolonging life even after terminal cancer has been diagnosed. It seeems that the use of behavior therapy can delay deaths from cancer and almost double the duration of survival.

Psychological Treatment in Cancer

Table 14 shows data from study to support this assertion (Grossarth-Maticek, 1980a). Twenty-four pairs of patients were formed who suffered from terminal cancer. They were matched on type of cancer, stage of growth, type of treatment, sex, and age; members of each pair were then allocated to treatment or control on a random basis. It will be seen that psychologically treated patients survived 5.07 years as compared with 3.09 years for controls.

In another study (Eysenck, 1988b; Grossarth-Maticek, 1980a), we studied 100 women suffering from terminal cancer of the breast. Half received chemotherapy, half did not; of these two groups, half received psychological therapy, half did not. Of those who received neither type of therapy, duration of survival was 11.28 months. Those who only had chemotherapy survived 14.08 months, while those who received only psychological therapy survived 14.92 months. Statistically, both effects are significant, but the combined effect (survival for 22.40 months) was significantly stronger than the simple addition of the two individual therapy effects would have suggested.

It is sometimes said that the results of behavior therapy in cancer and CHD, either prophylactically or in prolonging life, are too good to be true, yet much outside evidence supports the efficacy of different types of psychological therapy on cancer and CHD, some of which reports results even better than those described here. To take only the most recent study, Spiegel, Bloom, Kraemer, and Gottleib (1989) doubled the life expectancy of female patients with metastatic breast cancer, a result even better than similar studies reported by us (Eysenck, 1988a, 1988b). In the control group of Spiegel et al., life duration was 18.9 months, while in the therapy group it was 36.8 months. Such findings should be seen in the context of studies looking at the influence of psychosocial factors and interventions on the immune system—which presumably mediates the effects of life events, stress, and therapeutic psychological intervention—and on the occurrence

TABLE 14. Duration of survival of treated and control groups

Type of cancer	Number of pair of patients	Survival time, years		Sex	Age	
		Therapy group	Control group		Therapy	Control
Scrotal cancer	1	5.8	3.2+	M	34	35
Stomach cancer	1	4.8	1.8+	M	64	63
	2	2.4	2.3+	M	59	59
Bronchiolar	1	1.7	2.4−	M	42	42
	2	5.6	1.5+	M	59	60
	3	4.2	1.6+	M	60	60
	4	3.2	1.1+	M	47	46
	5	1.7	1.7=	M	39	39
	6	4.5	1.2+	M	58	58
	7	5.2	1.0+	M	63	64
Corpus uteri	1	6.8	4.2+	F	64	65
	2	4.5	4.8−	F	66	66
	3	7.2	3.5+	F	49	48
	4	8.2	3.1+	F	50	51
Cervical	1	5.5	4.2+	F	41	41
	2	6.1	4.0+	F	46	46
	3	3.2	3.3−	F	38	37
	4	4.5	4.1+	F	50	49
	5	2.8	3.6−	F	39	40
Colon and rectum carcinoma	1	9.5	4.2+	M	64	64
	2	7.5	2.1+	F	56	56
	3	6.3	4.9+	M	55	56
	4	4.8	4.3+	F	61	60
	5	5.7	4.1+	F	52	52
Total	24	5.07	3.09			

Note. Data from "Social Psychotherapy and Course of the Disease" by R. Grossarth-Maticek, 1980, *Psychotherapy and Psychosomatics*, *34*, p. 136.
Copyright 1980 by S. Karger.
Adapted by permission of the publisher and author.

and rigor of cancer. Before turning to a consideration of this evidence, it may be useful to consider studies suggesting the possibility of prophylactic intervention in CHD-prone probands.

Stress Management

Johnston (1989) has reviewed the literature in a very critical spirit but concludes that the evidence for the view that stress management may reduce CHD through the lowering of a large number of stress-related risk factors by moderate, or even small, amounts "is patchy, but a much stronger case can be made than would have seemed possible only ten years ago" (p. 277). The cautions optimism of this quotation is mainly based on the contributions of M. Friedman (1987); M. Friedman et al. (1984, 1986); Gill et al. (1985); Lovibond, Birrell, and Langeluddecke (1986); and Patel et al. (1985). Most convincing are the data presented by the recurrent coronary prevention project. If the results are less striking than those reported by Grossarth-Maticek, Eysenck, and Vetter (1988), this may be due to the fact that the validity of the type A concept is probably much lower than that of the Grossarth-Maticek type 2, that is, the CHD-prone type (Booth-Kewley & Friedman, 1987). It is also noteworthy that the theory linking stress with cancer and stress reduction with cancer survival has been elaborated much more convincingly (through the innervation of the immune system) than can be said of the relation between stress and stress management and CHD.

Bennett and Carroll (1990) similarly conclude a review of the evidence by saying that stress management techniques "not only reduce individual risk factors, they can also reduce mortality and morbidity to CHD" (p. 1). They also conclude that "risk factors combine multiplicatively, and small decreases on a number of risk factors may reduce the risk of CHD more than if only one risk factor is targeted (Johnston, 1989; D.A. Perkins, 1989), as in most medical interventions" (p. 81). These conclusions are very much in line with our own studies just detailed.

Finally, the conclusions drawn by Taylor (1990) in his review of health psychology, also support this view: "Research that examines whether or not psychological and social factors are involved in health and illness has largely made its point." (p. 46) He goes on to say that investigations have addressed the direct impact of stress and other psychological states on physiological processes, the impact of psychological and social factors on risky health practices, and the impact of psychological and social factors on how people respond to potential illness states, such as whether or not they engage in appropriate illness behavior. He concludes that the field has advanced to an unprecedented level of complexity in research investigations. . . . and that health psychology affords the opportunity to look beyond particular disorders to the broad principles of thought and behavior that cut across specializations of diseases or problems studied to elucidate more fundamental psychosocial mechanisms.

Some of the resulting complexities are illustrated in the work of Brown and McGill (1989) and Scheier et al. (1989). They highlighted the importance of optimism in the recovery of patients from coronary artery disease bypass surgery, demonstrating again the interaction of psychological states, personality, and medical illness or recovery. Brown and McGill demonstrated the complex interaction of personality traits such as optimism, which is closely linked with extraversion (Eysenck & Eysenck, 1985) and stress.

Positive life events are generally believed to have beneficial effects on health, but apparently this is only true when probands have a positive self-concept (optimism). Brown and McGill (1989) outline an identity-disruption model of stress, which holds that an accumulation of life events that are inconsistent with the self-concept leads to illness. Thus, positive life events in probands with a negative, pessimistic self-concept were predicted (and found) to predict the development of illness over time. Clearly, oversimplified concepts of "stress" may lead to erroneous predictions and may account for many failures to replicate in the literature.

The findings of Brown and McGill (1989) find support in an experimental study by Brebner (1990), who showed that introverts tend to generalize experiences of failure, extraverts experiences of success, thus developing pessimistic or optimistic personality traits. Brebner considers such generalization of failure experiences as an important form of stress, but of course, it is not usually mentioned in traditional stress inventories. It is noteworthy that the characteristics of cancer-prone probands agree to a considerable extent with those of introverts, while CHD probands tend to show more the characteristics of extraverts (Eysenck, 1990b). These apparent relationships between predisposition to disease and well-established personality types are well worth following up along theoretical and experimental lines.

One additional study that confirms the importance of an optimistic, extraverted attitude in mediating beneficial rather than negative health effects has looked at the effects of alcohol consumption, with special emphasis on the *reasons* for drinking (Grossarth-Maticek & Eysenck, in press-c). A group of 1,700 male subjects were tested and followed up for 13 years, when death and cause of death were established. A questionnaire administered at the beginning of the study served to classify drinkers as S-drinkers (drinking to drown their sorrows) or P-drinkers (drinking for pleasure, to celebrate success, for enjoyment). Stress or absence of stress was also noted on the basis of an interviewer-administered questionnaire. Results are shown in Table 15. The table shows that P-drinkers, with or without stress, have a lower mortality than nondrinkers, while S-drinkers, with or without stress, do significantly worse than nondrinkers. These results remain when level of drinking is controlled. It is quite likely that in studying the health effects of smoking, too, one should pay attention to the *reasons* for smoking (Eysenck, 1973; Spielberger, 1986); there might be a similar division there between those who smoke for pleasure and those who want to control their tenseness and anxiety. This is another area disregarded by adherents of present-day "orthodoxy."

Possibly also related to "optimism," and certainly to extraversion (Eysenck & Eysenck, 1985; is mobility (walking, jogging, athletics, sport), and here, too, there is evidence that sports are good for you. Grossarth-Maticek et al. (1990) have shown that people who are actively engaged in sports have enhanced longevity, as compared with people who are not so engaged. Worse off were those who started off in sport but gave up in middle age. It is noteworthy that in our therapy groups, there was a general tendency for probands after therapy to increase significantly participation

TABLE 15. Mortality of drinkers and abstainers as a function of stress and motivation for drinking

	With stress ($n = 203$) (%)		Without stress ($n = 201$) (%)	
No alcohol				
Cancer	25 (12.3)		8 (3.9)	
CHD	23 (11.3)		7 (3.4)	
Other causes				
of death	26 (12.8)		12 (5.9)	
Total	74 (36.5)		27 (13.4)	
Still living	129 (63.5)		174 (86.6)	

Alcohol Consumers	Pleasure drinkers $n = 191$ 27.4%		Sorrow drinkers $n = 506$ 72.6%		Pleasure drinkers $n = 481$ 79.5%		Sorrow drinkers $n = 124$ 20.5%	
		(27.4)		(72.6)		(79.5)		(20.5)
Cancer	18	(9.4)	87	(17.1)	23	(4.7)	11	(8.8)
CHD	11	(5.7)	59	(11.6)	12	(2.5)	7	(5.6)
Other causes								
of death	20	(10.4)	93	(18.3)	23	(4.7)	17	(13.7)
Total	49	(25.7)	239	(47.2)	58	(12.1)	35	(28.2)
Still living	142	(74.3)	267	(52.8)	423	(87.9)	89	(71.8)

CHD, coronary heart disease.
Note. Unpublished data, R. Grossarth-Maticek and H.J. Eysenck

in sports; there was no such tendency to give up smoking (Eysenck and Grossarth-Maticek, 1991).

A Causal Link Between Cancer and Personality

A brief outline may here be given of the way the connection between personality–stress and disease may be mediated by hormonal and physiological factors. A more detailed outline is given elsewhere (Eysenck, 1986). Figure 9 illustrates the assumed causal pathway. Personality (type 1) and stress combine and interact to produce feelings of helplessness, hopelessness, and depression; these in turn produce hormonal and other reactions of which cortisol is here given as the representative (others are the endogenous opiates, adrenocorticotropic hormone, etc.). These in turn produce immune deficiency, which allows budding cancers to develop. The well-established fact that immune reactions can be conditioned along classic lines suggests one possible way such reactions may be learned (Ader & Cohen, 1975; Solvason, Ghanta, & Hiramoto, 1988). A good deal of evidence supports such a model.

The model owes much to a similar one by Solomon (1985; Solomon, Levine, & Kraft, 1968; Solomon & Moos, 1964), who has argued powerfully for the concept of an "immunosuppression-prone" personality

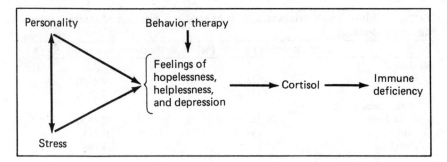

FIGURE 9. The assumed caused pathway whereby hormonal and physiological factors mediate the connection between personality, stress, and disease.

(Solomon, 1985). Having surveyed the literature, he produced first 35, and later another 30 postulates, many of which are relevant to this discussion. The main postulates of interest follow, numbered in sequence, i.e. differently from the way they are stated by him.

Solomon's Postulates (1987)

1. Enduring coping style and personality factors (trait characteristics) should influence the susceptibility of an individual's immune system to alteration by exogenous events, including reactions to events. (Thus, an "immunosuppression-prone" behavioral pattern is hypothesized.)
2. Emotional upset and distress (state characteristics) should alter the incidence, severity, and/or course of diseases that are immunologically resisted (infectious and neoplastic) or are associated with aberrant immunologic function (allergic and autoimmune).
3. Severe emotional disturbance and mental dysfunction should be accompanied by immunologic abnormalities.
4. Experimental behavioral manipulation (for example, stress, conditioning) should have immunologic consequences.
5. Experimental manipulation of appropriate parts of the central nervous system (CNS) should have immunologic consequences.
6. Hormones and other substances regulated or elaborated by the CNS should influence immune mechanisms.
7. Biochemical and functional similarities might be expected between the substances modulating the function and reactivity of the CNS (neuropeptides) and the substances with comparable effects on the immune system (cytokines).
8. Behavioral interventions (such as psychotherapy, relaxation techniques, imagery, biofeedback, and hypnosis) should be able to enhance or optimize immune function.

9. Altered CNS neurotransmitter receptor-site sensitivities believed to be associated with mental illnesses should be reflected in lymphocyte receptors.
10. The "functional" modes of expression of CNS and immune system should be similar.

Linn, Linn, and Jensen (1981) have shown that stress and anxiety are associated with depressed immunological response. Levy (1985) and Levy, Herberman, Lippman, and d'Angelo (1987) found that natural killer (NK) cell activity in breast cancer patients was strongly correlated with psychosocial stress indicators, which accounted for 51% of the baseline NK activity variance. Green and Green (1987) reported that relaxation increases salivary immunoglobin A1. Bandura, Cioffi, Taylor, and Brouillard (1988) found that perceived self-inefficacy in exercising control over cognitive stressors activated endogenous opioid systems. Kiecolt-Glaser, Rickers, et al. (1984) found that distressed and lonely probands had significantly higher cortisol levels and a lower level of NK cell activity. Glaser et al. (1986) discovered stress-related impairments in cellular immunity, and Glaser and Kiecolt-Glaser (1985) found that even "relatively mild stress" depressed cellular immunity in healthy adults. Kiecolt-Glaser, Rickers, et al. (1984) found that high scorers on stressful life events and loneliness had significantly lower levels of NK cell activity. Herberman (quoted in Solomon, 1985); Irwin, Vale, and Britton (1987); Nemeroff et al. (1984); and Rou, Rose, Sunderland, Moritisa, and Murphy (1988) found impaired immune reaction in depressed groups. Linn, Linn, and Klimas (1988); Arnetz et al. (1987); Glaser, Kiecolt-Glaser, Speicher, and Holliday (1985); and Shavit, Lewis, Terman, Gale, and Leibeskind (1989) found impaired immune reactions to stress. Jemmott and Magloire (1988) found that stress lowered salivary concentrations of S-IgA, while social support increased them. Grossarth-Maticek and Eysenck (1989b) found that behavior therapy significantly increased the percentage of lymphocytes in terminally ill women suffering from cancer and also increased their survival time. Pennebaker, Kiecolt-Glaser, and Glaser (1988) found that self-disclosure improved cellular immune functioning. Kiecolt-Glaser et al. (1985) found an enhancement of immunocompetence by relaxation and social contact.

Irwin, Daniels, Bloom, Smith, and Weiner (1987) have shown that life events can cause depression and can reduce the effectiveness of the immune function. Similarly, Murphy, Monson, Sobol, and Leighton (1987), in a prospective study of 1,003 adults, found a significant correlation between depression and mortality. Rodin (1984, 1986) showed that appropriate psychotherapy reduced depression *and* cortisol level through psychotherapy. Dabbs and Hopper (in press) showed that cortisol levels correlated with anxiety, depression, and high heart rate.

Of particular interest in relation to this theory are, of course, studies of cancer patients in which physiological treatment shows both improvement in psychological status and immune function when treatment patients are compared with control patients. Cousins (1989) summarizes one such study, which showed a significant decline in depression and psychological distress generally and a significant increase in "quality of life" scores; at the same time the functioning of the immune system exhibited significant improvement as shown by the number of immune cells in the NK cells family. (This of course is not necessarily a good index of immune functioning). A paper by Levy, Herberman, Lippman, and d'Angelo (1987) has already been mentioned, relating stress factors with sustained depression of NK cell activity, but equally important is another paper by Levy and her colleagues (Levy, Herberman, Maluish, Schlien, and Lippman, 1985) on prognostic risk assessment in primary breast cancer by behavioral and immunological parameters. They found that depressed cancer patients tend to have poorer NK-cell activity and greater likelihood of tumor spread. Also relevant is an article by Temoshok (1985), relating psychological and immune-system response to cutaneous malignant melanoma. She found that patients whose attitudes and emotions were active instead of passive exhibited better immune function and slower tumor spread.

Another relationship is between social support and immune function. Thus, in a community sample of the elderly, higher levels of social support were associated with total lymphocyte count and the ability of lymphocytes to subdivide when stimulated with mitogen (Thomas, Goodwin, & Goodwin, 1985.) Of particular interest is a quite recent study by Baron, Cutrona, Hicklin, Russell, and Lubaroff (1990), who investigated the effect of social support on immune functioning among spouses and cancer patients. They found that participants who had greater social support had faster T-cell proliferation when stimulated by the mitogen PHA and also were more effective in destroying target tumor cells in comparison with individuals who were below the median on reported social support. Neither the incidence of negative life events nor the existence of depressive symptoms were found to mediate this relation, but perhaps personality variables might have done so; the medium involved in producing these effects is at present unknown.

Pennebaker (1985, 1989) has described the way in which inhibition can be viewed as a chronic stressor, resulting in chronic autonomic and corticol arousal. This, in turn, leads to endocrinal activity that compromises the immune system, increasing susceptibility to disease. Pennebaker (1989) and his colleagues have reported that inhibiting one's desire to confide about traumatic events is associated with heightened electrodermal responding, decreased immunocompetence levels, and increase in disease. Other studies demonstrating the role of inhibitory mechanisms in decreased immune functions and in the development of disease (Cox & McKay, 1982; Jemmot, 1987) support this view, as does McClelland (1989).

Finally, the relationship between mood and the immune-system response has been established in a series of studies (e.g., Baker, 1987; Dillon & Baker, 1985–1986; Linn, Linn, & Jensen, 1984; McClelland, Floor, Davidson, & Saron, 1980; McClellon, Ross, & Patel, 1985; Stone, Cox, Valdimarsdottir, Jandorf, & Neale, 1987). Animal studies, too, have contributed to the formulation of the model (e.g., Borysenko & Borysenko, 1982; Glaser, Thorn et al., 1985; Laudenslager, Ryan, Drugan, Hyson, & Maier, 1983; and for a review, Justice, 1985.)

The studies cited are among only the most recent; for reviews of the older and perhaps less convincing material, the following are suggested: Antoni (1987); Baker (1987); Jemmott and Locke (1984); Kennedy, Kiecolt-Glaser, and Glaser (1988); Korneva, Klimenko, and Shkhinek (1985); N. Miller (1983, 1985); Plotnikoff, Faith, Murgo, and Good (1986); Steptoe (1989); and Teshina (1986). Taking all the published data together, they do seem to support the sort of model suggested by Eysenck (1986) Dilman and Ostroumova (1984), and Kanazir et al. (1984) and briefly outlined previously. There is evidence that (a) personality and stress produce immunodestructive substances in the bloodstream; (b) that these substances do have such an immunodestructive function, and that (c) behavioral manipulations can reverse this process. Thus, there appears to exist at least a preliminary model to explain along causal lines the effectiveness of behavior therapy in prophylaxis for cancer and in prolonging life in cancer sufferers.

There is one apparent objection to this argument. As Zonderman, Costa, and McCrae (1989) have shown, there is no evidence in a nationally representative sample for any correlation between depressive symptoms and cancer morbidity. The answer to this is very simple. Depression is a multifaceted set of symptoms, like fever, which may have diverse causes and relate to different disorders; the difference between reactive and endogenous depression is perhaps the best known. The type of depression referred to in the theory discussed here is subclinical and might be defined as "hopelessness depression" (Alloy, Abramson, Metalsky, & Hartlage, 1988). This concept is largely based on the work of Seligman (1975) and L.Y. Abramson, Seligman, and Teasdale (1978) and is essentially a cognitive diathesis-stress theory of depression (Alloy, Clements, & Kolden, 1985). According to this theory, "a proximal sufficient cause of depression is an expectation that highly desired outcomes are unlikely to occur, or that highly aversive outcomes are likely to occur, and that no response in one's repertoire will change the likelihood of occurrence of these outcomes" (Alloy et al., 1988, p. 7). It is in this sense that the term has been used in our research. Other varieties of depression may or may not be relevant, and it is important to note that animal work has also emphasized the importance of differentiating between escapable and inescapable shocks and the vital contribution of predictability (S.M. Miller, 1981).

CHD and Sclerosis: Psychological Therapy Effects

As far as CHD is concerned, there is less material to review, but sclerosis is an obvious intermediary. Grossarth-Maticek, Eysenck, Gallasch, Vetter, and Frentzel-Beyme (in press) have reported a study in which 100 cancer-prone and 92 CHD-prone probands had the degree of sclerosis in the fundus of the eye measured on a 3-point scale by a leading ophthalmologist; before and after therapy (for a randomly selected 50% of probands in each case) and at similar points of time for probands in the control group. Figure 10 shows the results. Type 2 probands had significantly *higher* levels of sclerosis than type 1 probands, and the therapy group had a significantly *lower* degree of sclerosis; more so for CHD-prone type 2 than for cancer-prone type 1 probands. This experiment is in urgent need of replication.

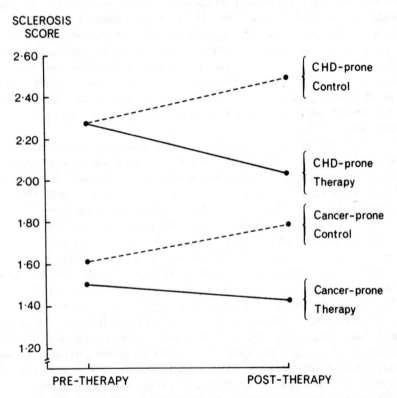

FIGURE 10. Sclerosis in cancer-prone and coronary heart disease-prone probands and effects of behavior therapy Heidelberg study. (*Note.* From "Changes in Degree of Sclerosis as a Function of Prophylactic Treatment in Cancer-Prone and CHD-Prone Probands" by R. Grossarth-Maticek, H.J. Eysenck, B. Gallasch, H. Vetter, and R. Frentzel-Beyme, in press, *Behaviour Research and Therapy.* Copyright 1991 by H.J. Eysenck. Reprinted by permission.)

It is of course necessary to preserve caution in interpreting the results shown in Figure 10. As in the case of epidemiology generally, there are no singular causes producing single results. Thus, Cobb and Rose (1973) showed that air traffic controllers have a higher incidence of hypertension than controls and produce the condition at a younger age. This could be interpreted as a direct effect of the greater stress under which air traffic controllers work. Hypertension, however, is strongly related to alcohol consumption in air traffic controllers (De Frank, Jenkins, & Rose, 1987). It is possible that the drinking may be the important determinant, because alcohol intake is known to raise blood pressure (MacMahon, 1987). Complications of this kind are the rule in this field, rather than the exception.

Clearly, the Grossarth-Maticek and Eysenck data concerning the prophylactic effects of behavior therapy for cancer and CHD are equally subject to this caution. We have shown (Grossarth-Maticek et al., in press) that after therapy there is a very significant shift from type 1 or type 2 behavior to type 4 behavior; there is no change in smoking habits. As Pearl (1925) has pointed out, however, there is a life-style that embraces many different behavior patterns, and changing one may change many others, one of which, or any combination of which, can carry the burden of changes in cancer proneness or CHD proneness. Research is only at the beginning of the scientific study of these complex nomological networks and should not pretend to a greater or more secure understanding of these causal effects than in reasonable under the circumstances.

In Eysenck (1990a), I have discussed the social implications of this type of work. Clearly, preventive medicine is much more humane in its consequences, as well as much cheaper, than traditional medicine, which waits until the disease has manifested itself before attempting any intervention. Many practical, social, and ethical problems are raised when one considers the possibility of introducing methods of this kind for the prevention of cancer and CHD into the social systems at present concerned with health, but it is time that the issues were taken seriously and debated in a meaningful fashion.

What is most important from the point of view of this book, of course, is the demonstration of the heightened probability of a *causal* relation between stressed personality and cancer and CHD. The failure to demonstrate such a relationship between smoking and disease, shown in previous chapters is the most vulnerable point in the orthodox view. These results show that it may be possible to demonstrate causal relations following accepted scientific methodology and to establish personality and stress as important risk factors in cancer and CHD.

8
Summary and Conclusions

In spite of all the criticisms that may justifiably be made of modern epidemiological methods and findings, it is possible to make some fairly definitive statements that characterize the present status of research in the field covered by this book.

1. It is clear beyond doubt that there is a debate concerning risk factors in cancer and coronary heart disease (CHD), particularly smoking. On the one hand is a large group of physicians, epidemiologists, and others who claim that smoking is the major cause of cancer and CHD and that if only we could stop people smoking, large numbers of lives could be saved. On the other hand is a large number of physicians, epidemiologists, oncologists, and other scientists who believe that these diseases involve a multiplicity of risk factors, interacting in complex ways, of which smoking is only one, and not by any means the most important. The media have almost entirely suppressed representation of this alternative view and have given rise to the completely unjustified and unscientific belief that smoking is the main and almost the only risk factor for cancer and CHD. It seems about time that the truth regarding the existence of this debate be publicly acknowledged and that the usual exaggerations concerning the effects of smoking cease to be published and broadcast.

2. There is now little doubt that smoking has certain positive effects that account for its popularity and for the curious fact that even people who believe that smoking causes disease still continue to smoke. Among the positive features of smoking, which have now been firmly established by research, (O'Connor & Stravynski, 1982) are its ability to raise the cortical arousal level and thus counteract boredom and fatigue; its ability to make anxious and tense persons relax, thus reducing the impact of negative emotions; and its power to increase attention and vigilance, thus enabling people to work longer and harder, and more efficiently, than they could do otherwise. These are important advantages, which should be set against the disadvantages of smoking. There does not seem to be any truth in the allegation that smoking is an addiction, even if that term could be defined

in such a way as to have a scientific meaning. People maintain the smoking habit because of the positive effects of smoking on their psychological well-being; if one substitutes alternative behaviors that serve the same needs, smoking can readily be given up as being no longer required.

3. The relative importance of smoking as a risk factor, compared with psychosocial and other risk factors, has received a good deal of attention. Roughly speaking, (Grossarth-Maticek, Eysenck, & Vetter, 1988) personality and stress appear to be six times as important as smoking in the statistical correlation between disease and risk factors. (Replication of this study is, of course, an urgent necessity; single findings may be subject to undiscovered errors.) This does not mean that smoking is in any way harmless, but it certainly puts into perspective its possible influence on cancer and CHD.

4. What emerges with particular clarity from all the work that has been summarized in these pages is the importance of psychosocial factors, that is, stress and the individual's reaction to stress (Eysenck, 1988b). Of all the risk factors considered, this is perhaps the most important, showing the strongest correlation with death from cancer and CHD. It is curious, considering the 2,000-year history of theories concerning psychosocial factors, that the medical profession has, on the whole, failed to pay much attention to the importance of stress and personality in the causation of disease and tends to reject claims that stress is a real killer. The evidence is too strong now to reject such claims out of hand.

5. The only model that may be adequate to contain the known facts in this field is a multifactorial synergistic model, that is, one including many risk factors and in which these risk factors act in a synergistic (i.e., multiplicative) rather than in an additive fashion. Thus, in our own work, smoking has always been found not to be strongly correlated with cancer or with CHD in groups where there was no stress or where a healthy personality counteracted the stress and managed to cope with it. Positive correlations with disease do appear strongly in populations of type 1 or 2, that is, populations where stress is endemic and coping behavior is inadequate.

6. So far I have discussed only correlations between risk factors such as smoking, stress, personality, and so on, and disease; it is well known that correlation does not imply causation and that statistical association may suggest but does not prove causation. The best demonstration that a causal model may be indicated is furnished by intervention studies. As I have shown, the evidence does not suggest that quitting smoking affects cancer or CHD much. Where quitters are self-selected, they already differ profoundly in their state of health from continuing smokers, and any differences in outcome are more likely to be due to this difference than to the effects of quitting. When quitters are part of a therapy group, their future health does not differ, or differs only slightly, from that of continuing smokers. The evidence is confused at best, but it certainly does not support

the widely publicized claims that have been made for the beneficial effects of quitting smoking.

7. The position is quite different with respect to psychosocial factors, for which the evidence now seems quite strong that the application of the methods of behavior therapy to people suffering from stress and inadequate coping mechanisms can prevent cancer and CHD, when groups receiving such help are compared with groups not receiving it. Thus, not only are psychosocial factors statistically much more closely related to disease, but there is evidence for a causal influence here that is absent in the case of smoking (Eysenck & Grossarth-Maticek, 1991).

8. Clearly, there must be intermediary factors intervening between stress–personality and disease, and the discovery of such factors is one of the major tasks for future research. It seems reasonable to assume that the major intermediary in the case of cancer is the immune system, and there is evidence that behavior therapy can improve the efficacy of the immune system, while stress has the opposite effect (Eysenck, 1986; Rodin, 1984, 1986). Similarly, there is evidence for a marked influence of stress and behavior therapy on the degree of sclerosis shown by individual probands (Grossarth-Maticek et al., in press). With this whole field of research being so young, this area has not been sufficiently researched to reach any definite conclusion, but these are suggestions that are certainly worth following up.

It would not be right to pretend that the position of this research is a very comfortable one, or that the knowledge is as adequate to the challenges of disease as it ought to be. One of the major reasons for this unsatisfactory position is that research money has gone to areas that have proved unrewarding, e.g. The Multiple Risk Factor Intervention Trial.

In particular, research is vital in the area least investigated, namely, the effects of stress and of behavior therapy on the immune system. Prospective studies of the kind pioneered by Grossarth-Maticek (see references) should be repeated with the inclusion of direct measures of immune system assays and with multiple measures of sclerosis. Only in this way, will researchers achieve greater knowledge of the causes of cancer and CHD and of the most efficient methods of preventing them. As Kurt Lewin used to say: "There is nothing as practical as a good theory." No such theory is likely to arise from the simple repetition of the saying that "smoking causes cancer and CHD." What is required is a theory that incorporates all that is known about the complex interaction between the many risk factors involved, the synergistic way in which they multiply their effects, and the way in which intervention does or does not act to prevent cancer and CHD in cancer-prone and CHD-prone persons. Researchers now have a good idea about the direction research should take, and it seems obvious that psychological factors play too large and important a part to be neglected, as they usually have been in the past. If prevention is better than (doubtful) cure, then the neglect of psychological factors in disease becomes irresponsible. This is the direction in which research should go if researchers really want to save lives and prevent cancer and CHD.

The outlines of a general theory here suggested may be worthy of direct experimentation to support or disprove it; it seems the only way to reconcile apparently contradictory findings. What is suggested is that the biological effects of smoking follow a negatively accelerated growth curve, whose asymptote depends on the number of cigarettes smoked per day but that ceases to grow beyond a relatively short period of 1 or 2 years and whose symptote is not influenced to any appreciable degree by further smoking or cessation of smoking. These biological effects have little direct influence on the initiation of cancer or CHD but interact synergistically with other risk factors like genetic predisposition, stress, personality, drinking, and so on. This synergistic interaction suggests why psychological intervention is such a powerful factor in preventing cancer and CHD and even in prolonging life in terminally ill cancer patients. Such intervention removes not an additive but a multiplicative risk factor, hence, having a disproportionate effect on the total sum of risk factors.

Omitting smoking does no have any such effect becuase it does not alter the height of the asymptote, which determines the biological effects of smoking on the organism, in so far as these are relevant to cancer and CHD. This suggests that possibly the main action of smoking is a catalyst, increasing the effects of other risk factors. The facts certainly fit the model, but clearly, many more deductions need to be tested and confirmed before the theory can be accepted as a valid picture of what is happening in this extremely complex system of interacting variables. Inevitably, many anomalies, contradictions, and puzzles remain; these are present in any scientific theory and demand theory-directed reserch to clear a way; even Newton's theory of gravitation was beset by anomalies for hundreds of years.

9
Epilogue

The question of risk factors for cancer and coronary heart disease (CHD) and the relative importance of smoking as a risk factor are clearly important scientific problems that should be solved by the use of traditional scientific methods. Yet, conclusions have often been based on inadequate methodology, doubtful assumptions, inappropriate statistics, and inadmissible extrapolations.

In this, the whole controversy resembles similar controversies that have raged around issues like the role of cholesterol in CHD or that of fluoridation of the water supply. In both cases, publicity campaigns were waged to get people to substitute margarine for butter, change the whole diet to lower cholesterol levels, increase the fluoride level of the water supply, and quite generally change people's habits in line with supposititious benefits to their health. Had these benefits been real, and had these changes in fact produced better health and long life, the support given these measures might be understandable. However, as already noted, apparently few obvious benefits are derived from a low-cholesterol diet, and in fact it might be linked with increasing risks of cancer.

I cannot pronounce on these developments as far as their medical background is concerned; the new developments may have as little substance as the old. They may, however, have the beneficial effect of making lay readers, and possibly even medical readers, less prone to take too seriously any pronouncements of epidemiological experts based on insufficient evidence and possibly defective studies. What is being criticized is not the individual scientist who draws the wrong conclusion from his data, or who commits errors of one kind or another in his experimental methodology or in his statistical analysis. To err is human, and all scientists are prone to blunders of one kind or another. But scientists should be modest in their claims, should refuse to exaggerate the certainty of their conclusions, and should always be open to correction and the consideration of contrary evidence. In particular, they should refrain from advocating far-reaching social actions on the basis of doubtful, fallible, disputed, and insufficient evidence.

The exaggerated claims concerning the degree of risks attending cigarette smoking in the causation of cancer and CHD must stand with the exaggerated claims concerning cholesterol as a warning to scientists to avoid prematurely advocating social action. As Claude Bernard warned a hundred years ago: "In ignorance, abstain!"

One additional matter requires discussion in this context. The premature claims for the preventive possibilities of a reduced cholesterol diet in relation to CHD, and giving up smoking in relation to cancer and CHD, and the widespread publicity these have received through the media, have suggested to the layman that a far greater certitude attends to these claims than can be justified scientifically, as discussed. The recent findings that these claims may very well be in fact unfounded, and that indulgence in a low-cholesterol diet may in fact harm rather than benefit the individual, have led to bewilderment and a feeling, only too well justified, that expert opinion on medical matters may sometimes the untrustworthy and that the constant reversals of recommendations for a healthier living emanating from such sources indicate a lack of true knowledge. As Le Fanu (1987) has pointed out, in 1930s, nutritionists advised us to eat more eggs and butter and drink more milk. A few years later, all these nutriments became anathema, in the interests of a low-cholesterol diet. now, we are told that this was all a mistake, that there is no harm in eggs, butter, and milk, and that they may even be good for us. Clearly, something has gone wrong when opposite recommendations are made on the apparent basis of "scientific" evidence, and the public has a right to be bewildered and to doubt if such advice is really based on fact rather than passing fancy. This may undermine public faith in the objectivity of science and the truth-value of scientists' published beliefs; it is, indeed, the old story of the boy who cried "Wolf." Having cried wolf so often only to retract the statements of the alleged danger, nutritionists, epidemiologists, and other medical specialists are now in danger of being disbelieved even when their warnings are only too well justified. Worse yet, warnings that are not justified by the state of our present knowledge may themselves increase stress and lead to very serious health consequences. My study with Grossarth-Maticek (Grossarth-Maticek & Eysenck, 1989a) has shown that such fears may very well be only too real and that the constantly repeated media threat that smoking kills may in fact become a self-fulfilling prophecy!

When the assertions made by apparently authoritative bodies and persons, such as the Royal College of Physicians or the Surgeon General of the United States, would seem to exaggerate the consequences of smoking in deaths from cancer and CHD and the virtues of giving up smoking, it is small wonder that the media, as well as politicians, take up the chorus, not realizing that there is little justification for the claims made, and that these assertions have received damaging criticisms from leading oncologists, immunologists, and other scientists.

The only responsible way out of this impasse, is to return to the precepts that have always guided science. Publications should contain not only assertions of position, based on selected evidence, but should deal fairly and squarely with all objections, criticisms, and contrary findings. Conclusions should be justified by the evidence and carefully qualified rather than extreme in their certainly when this is not warranted. Finally, no publicity should be given to results, and no publication urged or taken, unless there is virtual agreement among experts (as there most certainly is not in relation to the effects of smoking) about the issue in question. Even then the fallibility of research in such very complex areas should be emphasized and the possibility of error acknowledged. These are the ways science has progressed and has acquired its unique prestige.

In this area, politics has taken over from science, to a dangerous degree. Consider the tactics that have been used widely in connection with the "smoking causes disease" issue. It has become difficult for those who wish to examine the problem objectively to obtain research funds or to publish their data, if they are not in line with official policy. Newspapers refuse to discuss the facts objectively and pretend that unanimity exists when in reality confusion reigns, and criticism of the "orthodox" view is widespread. Alternative models are dismissed without proper examination and are seldom mentioned in official publications. Investigators who show an interest in such models encounter obstacles in their careers and may have all support withdrawn, regardless of the quality of their research. These are not conditions that encourage high-quality scientific research, and it is small wonder that the field is confused and full of anomalies. In this book, I have tried to set out the facts as carefully and objectively as possible and to point out the major conclusions that may be drawn.

The failure of many workers in this field to be objective and to tell the public fairly and squarely about the present position of research has been exposed most convincingly by Effron (1984) in her book on *The Apocalyptics*, which cuts a much wider swath than the present book, but which justifies amply its subtitle: *Cancer and the Big Lie*. It deals with "the ideological corruption of cancer research in the United States." The author contends, and demonstrates, that an extreme environmental movement, which she calls "the apocalyptics," has politically distorted research in environmental cancer, saturating the United States with theories of cancer that are pure myths. Her book should be read by all concerned with the problem of cancer origin and propagation; the problem considered in this book is only one facet of this much wider phenomenon. There is no doubt that smoking is one of many risk factors in cancer and CHD, but the notion that it is all important, and that reduction in smoking would have far-reaching benevolent consequences as far as cancer and CHD are concerned, is just one of those myths that Effron castigates.

Much remains obscure, but some features of the scene must be regarded as hopeful. If stress and other psychosocial factors are indeed killers, it does seem that suitable prophylactic means are at hand to delay or prevent cancer and CHD. Behavior therapy is a very cheap and convenient way of safeguarding healthy probands from cancer and CHD, and from every point of view, prevention must be better than largely nonexistent cures or very expensive treatments with often disastrous side-effects. If only researchers could abandon the present unhealthy preoccupation with smoking and focus on all the risk factors involved, including stress, hereditary predisposition and so on, we might in reality save all those lives that a well-intentioned but possibly misleading effort has tried to persuade us could be saved if only people gave up smoking. This is a serious issue, vital for hundreds of thousands of people, and we should not continue with a bland and biased disregard of the true facts of the case.

Am I being too positive in arguing for the importance of personality and psychologiocal factors in contributing to increased longevity? A recent study (Cousins, 1989) of 649 American oncologists, who reported their opinions on the importance of various psychosocial factors, suggests that the views here advocated are becoming quite widely accepted. A positive approach to the challenge of the illness was regarded as very or moderately important by 80%; a strong will to live, by 79%; emotional support from friends and family members, by 75%; the patient's ability to cope with stress, by 73%; the patient's involvement in creative and meaningful activities, by 63%; and strong religious or spiritual conviction, by 49%. Equally, the survey emphasized the doctor's duty in encouraging the patient to develop an attitude of hope and optimism concerning treatment outcome (95%), and providing referral to psychological counselling services (57%).

These data (Cousins, 1989) suggest a very enlightened attitude of specialists with respect to the importance of psychological factors in disease. It is curious that there is little evidence of a similarly enlightened attitude on the part of epidemiologists. To many readers only familiar with the writings of epidemiologists, the message of this book may sound unorthodox and even revolutionary; as the data quoted suggest, the message is widely accepted by specialists. Personality and psychological factors such as stress are of fundamental importance as risk factors for disease; no research worth the name can given meaningful results unless such factors are incorporated firmly within it. Causes of diseases such as cancer and CHD are not unitary but complex and varied, interacting in intricate and convoluted fashion; much remains to be discovered in this field before researchers can be sure of the facts. When researchers clearly can no longer do is to pretend that a single factor, such as smoking, is solely responsible for the tragedy of cancer and CHD.

References

Abelin, T. (1988). *Rauchen und Gesundheit*. Zurich: Schweizerische Vereinigung gegen Tuberkulose und Lungen Krankheiten.

Abramson, J.H., Sacks, U.I., & Cabana, E. (1971). Death certificate data as an indication of the presence of certain common diseases at death. *Journal of Chronic Diseases*, *14*, 417–431.

Abramson, L.Y., Seligman, M.E.P., & Teasdale, H. (1978). Learned helplessness in humans? Critique and reformulation. *Journal of Abnormal Psychology*, *87*, 49–74.

Ader, R., & Cohen, N. (1975). Behaviorally conditioned immuno-suppression. *Psychosomatic Medicine*, *37*, 333–340.

Aeberhardt, E. (Ed.). (1989). *Bericht zur Krebsverhütung*. Winterthur, Switzerland: E. Aeberhardt Stiftung.

Alloy, L.B., Abramson, L.Y., Metalsky, C., & Hartlage, S. (1988). The hopelessness theory of depression: Attributional aspects. *British Journal of Clinical Psychology*, *27*, 5–21.

Alloy, L.B., Clements, C., & Kolden, G. (1985). The cognitive diathesis—Stress theories of depression: Therapeutic implications. In S. Reiss & R. Bortzin (Eds.), *Theoretical issues in behavior therapy*. New York: Academic Press.

Allred, K.D., & Smith. T.W. (1989). The hardy personality: Cognitive and physiological responses to evaluate threat. *Journal of Personality and Social Psychology*, *56*, 257–266.

American Psychiatric Association (1980). *Diagnostic and statistical manual of mental disorders* (3rd ed.). Washington, DC: American Psychiatric Assocation.

Antoni, M.H. (1987). Neuroendocrine influences in psychoimmunology and neoplasia: A review. *Psychology and Health*, *1*, 3–24.

Arnetz, B., Wasserman, J., Petrini, B., Brenner, F., Levi, L., Eneroth, P., Solovaara, H., Hjelm, D., Thoerell, T., & Pettersen, I. (1987). Immune function in unemployed women. *Psychosomatic Medicine*, *49*, 3–12.

Ashton, H., & Stepney, R. (1982). *Smoking, psychology and pharmacology*. London: Tavistock.

Atteslander, P. (Ed.). (1989). *Smoking and mortality in Switzerland*. Zurich: Arbeitsgruppe Gesundheitsforschung.

Aviado, D.M. (1986). Health issues relating to "passive" smoking. In R.D. Tollison (Ed.), *Smoking and society* (pp. 137–166). Toronto: Lexington Books.

Baalen, D. van, & de Vries, M.J. (1987). *"Spontaneous" regression of cancer.* Rotterdam, The Netherlands: Erasmus University.

Baker, G.H.B. (1987). Psychological factors and immunity. *Journal of Psychosomatic Research, 31,* 1–10.

Baltrusch, H., Stangel, W., & Waltz, M. (1988). Cancer from the behavioral perspective: The Type C pattern. *Activitas Nervosa Superior, 30,* 18–20.

Bammer, K., & Newberry, B.H. (Eds.). (1981). *Stress and cancer.* Toronto: C.J. Hogrefe.

Bandura, A., Cioffi, D., Taylor, C.B., & Brouillard, M.E. (1988). Perceived self-efficacy in coping wth cognitive stressors and opioid activation. *Journal of Personality and Social Psychology, 55,* 479–488.

Baron, R.S., Cutrona, C.E., Hicklin, D., Russell, D.W., & Lubaroff, D.A. (1990). Social support and immune functions among spouses of cancer patients. *Journal of Personality and Social Psychology, 59,* 344–352.

Bauer, F.W., & Robbins, S.L. (1972). An autopsy study of cancer patients. *Journal of American Medical Assocaition, 227,* 1431–1474.

Beadenkopff, W.G., Abrams, M., Daoud, A., & Marks, R.U. (1963). An assessment of certain medical aspects of death certificate data for epidemiologic study of arteriosclerotic heart disease. *Journal of Chronic Disease, 16,* 249–262.

Beek, H.J. van. (no date). *Linguistic differences in the speech of cancer and CHD-patients.* Rotterdam: Erasmus University.

Belcher, J.R. (1971). World-wide differences in the sex ratio of bronchial carcinoma. *British Journal of Diseases of the Chest, 65,* 205–221.

Bennett, P., & Carroll, D. (1990). Stress management approaches to the prevention of coronary heart disease. *British Journal of Clinical Psychology, 29,* 1–12.

Berkson, J. (1958). Smoking and lung cancer: some observations in two recent reports. *Journal of the American Statistical Association, 53,* 28–38.

Berkson, J., & Elveback, L. (1960). Competing exponential risks, with particular reference to the study of smoking and lung cancer. *Journal of the American Statistical Association, 291,* 415–428.

Berridge, V., & Edwards, G. (1987). *Opium and the people: Opiate use in nineteenth century England.* New York: Yale University Press.

Binik, Y.M. (1985). Psychosocial prediction of sudden death: A reivew and critique. *Social Science and Medicine, 20,* 667–680.

Booth-Kewley, S., & Friedman, H. (1987). Psychological predictors of heart disease: A quantitative review. *Psychological Bulletin, 101,* 343–362.

Borysenko, M., & Borysenko, J. (1982). Stress, behavior and immunity: Animal models and mediating mechanisms. *General Hospital Psychiatry, 4,* 59–67.

Brebner, J. (1990). Personality and generalization as a source of stress. In J. Sarason, C. Spielberger, J. Strelau, & J. Brebner (Eds.), *Stress and anxiety* (Vol. 13, pp. 45–61). Washington, DC: Hemisphere.

Briggs, R.L. (1975). Quality of death certificate diagnosis as compared with autopsy findings. *Arizona Medicine, 32,* 617–624.

Brindley, D.N., & Rolland, Y. (1989). Possible connections between stress, diabetes, obesity, hypertension and altered lipoprotein metabolism that may result in atherosclerosis. *Clinical Science, 77,* 453–461.

Britton, M. (1974). Diagnostic errors discovered at autopsy. *ACTA Medica Scandinavica, 1696,* 203–210.

Brown, G.W., & Harris, T. (1978). Social origins of depression: A reply. *Psychological Medicine, 8,* 577–588.

Brown, J.D., & McGill, K.L. (1989). The cost of good fortune: When positive life events produce negative health consequences. *Journal of Personality and Social Psychology, 57,* 1103–1110.

Brownlee, K.A. (1965). A review of "Smoking and Health." *Journal of the American Statistical Association, 60,* 722–739.

Burch, P.R.J. (1976). *The biology of cancer: A new approach.* Lancaster: Medical and Technical Publishers.

Burch, P.R.J. (1978). Smoking and lung cancer: The problem of inferring cause. *Journal of the Royal Statistical Society, 141,* 437–477.

Burch, P.R.J. (1983). The Surgeon-General's "epidemiologic criteria for causality": A critique. *Journal of Chronic Diseases, 36,* 821–836.

Burch, P.R.J. (1986). Can epidemiology become a rigorous science? How big is The Big Kill? *IRCS Medical Science, 14,* 956–961.

Cameron, M., & McGoogan, E. (1981). A prospective study of 1152 hospital autopsies. Part I: Inaccuracies in death certificates. *Journal of Pathology, 133,* 273–283.

Cameron, M., & McGoogan, E. (1981). A prospective study of 1152 hospital autopsies: 2. Analysis of inaccuracies in clinical diagnoses and their significance. *Journal of Pathology, 134,* 285–300.

Chan, W.C., Colbourne, M.J., Fung, S.C., & Ho, H.C. (1979). Bronchial cancer in Hong Kong, 1976–1977. *British Journal of Cancer, 39,* 182–192.

Clark, S. (Ed.). (1989). *Smoke out: How the quality pressures the smoking debate.* London: Centre for Media Research and Analysis.

Cobb, S., & Rose, R.M. (1973). Hypertension, peptic ulcer and diabetes in air traffic controllers. *Journal of American Medical Association, 224,* 489–492.

Collins, R., Peto, R.R., MacMahon, S., Herbert, P., Fieback, V., Eberlein, K., Godwin, J., Qizilbash, N., Taylor, J., & Hennekens, C. (1990). Blood pressure, stroke, and coronary heart disease. *Lancet, 335,* 827–838.

Cooper, C.L. (1983). *Stress research.* New York: Wiley & Sons.

Cooper, C.L. (Ed.) (1989). *Psychosocial stress and cancer.* New York: John Wiley & Sons.

Cousins, N. (1989). *Head first: The biology of hope.* New York: Dutton.

Cox, D.R. (1970). *Analysis of binary data.* London: Chapman and Hall.

Cox, T., & McKay, C. (1982). Psychosocial factors and psychophysiological mechanisms in the aetiology and development of cancer. *Social Science and Medicine, 16,* 381–396.

Curwen, M.P., Kanaway, E.L., & Kanaway, N.G. (1954). The incidence of cancer of the lung and larynx in urban and rural districts. *British Journal of Cancer, 8,* 181–198.

Dabbs, J.M., & Hopper, C.H. (in press). Cortisol, arousal, and personality in two groups of normal men. *Personality & Individual Differences.*

Darrock, J.V. (1974). Multiplicative and additive interaction in contingency tables. *Biometrika, 61,* 207–214.

Dawber, T.R. (1980). *The Framingham study: The epidemiology of atherosclerotic disease.* Cambridge, MA: Harvard University Press.

Day, S.B. (Ed.). (1987). *Cancer, stress and death.* New York: Plenum.

De Frank, R.S., Jenkins, C.D. & Rose, R.M. (1987). A longitudinal investigation of the relationship among alcohol consumption, psychosocial factors and blood pressure. *Psychosomatic Medicine, 49*, 236–249.

Dembrowski, T.M. (1984). Stress and substance interaction effects on risk factors and reactivity. *Behavioral Medical Update, 6*, 16–19.

de Silva, P., & Eysenck, S.B.G. (1987). Personality and addictiveness in anorexia and bulimic patients. *Personality & Individual Differences, 8*, 749–751.

Dillon, K.M., & Baker, K.H., (1985–1986). Positive emotional states and enhancement of the immune system. *International Journal of Psychiatry and Medicine, 15*, 13–18.

Dilman, V.M., & Ostroumova, M.V. (1984). Hypothalamic, metabolic, and immune mechanisms of the influence of stress. In B.N. Fox & B.H. Newberry (Eds.), *Impact of psychoendocrine systems in cancer and immunity*. New York: C.J. Hogrefe.

Doll, R., & Peto, R. (1976). Mortality in relation to smoking: 20 years' observations of male British doctors. *British Medical Journal, 2*, 1525–1536.

Eaves, L.J., Eysenck, H.J., & Martin, N. (1989). *Genes, culture and personality*. New York: Academic Press.

Effron, E. (1984). *The apocalyptics: Cancer and the big lie*. New York: Simon & Schuster.

Enstrom, J.E. (1980). Cancer mortality among Mormons in California during 1968–1975. *Journal of the National Cancer Institute, 65*, 1073–1082.

Everitt, B.G. (1977). The Analysis of contingency tables. London: Chapman & Hall.

Everitt, B.S., & Smith, A.M.R. (1979). Interactions in contigency tables: A brief discussion of alternative definitions.

Eylenbosch, W.J., Depoorter, M., & Larebeke, N.V. (1988). *Primary prevention of cancer* (Vol. 19). New York: Raven Press.

Eysenck, H.J. (1965). *Smoking, health and personality*. London: Weidenfeld & Nicolson.

Eysenck, H.J. (1973). Personality and the maintenance of the smoking habit. In W.L. Dunn (Ed.), *Smoking behaviour: Motives and incentives*. Washington, DC: Winston/Wiley.

Eysenck, H.J. (1980). *The causes and effects of smoking*. London: Maurice Temple Smith.

Eysenck, H.J. (1984). Meta-analysis: An abuse of research integration. *Journal of Special Education, 18*, 41–59.

Eysenck, H.J. (1985). Personality, cancer and cardiovascular disease: A causal analysis. *Personality & Individual Differences, 5*, 535–557.

Eysenck, H.J. (1986). Smoking and Health. In R.D. Tollison (Ed.), *Smoking and society* (pp. 17–88). Lexington, MA: Lexington Books.

Eysenck, H.J. (1987). *Rauchen und Gesundheit*. Düsseldorf: W. Rau Verlag.

Eysenck, H.J. (1988a). Behavior therapy as an aid in the prevention of cancer and coronary heart disease. *Scandinavian Journal of Behavior Therapy, 17*, 171–188.

Eysenck, H.J. (1988b). The respective importance of personality, cigarette smoking and interaction effects for the genesis of cancer and coronary heart disease. *Personality & Individual Differences, 9*, 453–464.

Eysenck, H.J. (1989). Prevention of cancer and coronary heart disease and the reduction in the cost of the National Health Service. *Journal of Social, Political & Economic Studies, 14*(1), 25–47.

Eysenck, H.J. (1990a). The prediction of death from cancer by means of personality/stress questionnaire: Too good to be true? *Perceptual and Motor Skills, 71*, 216–218.

Eysenck, H.J. (1990b). Type A behavior and coronary heart disease: The third stage. *Journal of Social Behavior & Personality, 5*, 25–44.

Eysenck, H.J., & Eysenck, M.W. (1985). *Personality and individual differences.* New York: Plenum.

Eysenck, H.J., & Grossarth-Maticek, R. (1991). Creative novation behaviour therapy as a prophylactic treatment for cancer and coronary heart disease: 2. Effects of treatment. *Behaviour Research and Therapy., 29*, 17–31.

Eysenck, H.J., & Martin, I. (Eds.). (1987). *Theoretical foundations of behavior therapy.* New York: Plenum.

Eysenck, H.J., & O'Connor, K. (1979). Smoking, arousal and personality. In A. Remond & C. Izard (Eds.), *Electrophysical effects of nicotine* (pp. 34–43). Amsterdam, The Netherlands: Elsevier/North Holland.

Eysenck, H.J., Tarrant, M., & Woolf, M. (1960). Smoking and personality. *British Medical Journal, 1*, 1456–1460.

Feistein, A.R. (1988). Scientific standards in epidemiologic studies of the menace of daily life. *Science*, December 1257–1263.

Feinstein, A.R., & Wells, C.K. (1974). Cigarette smoking and lung cancer: The problem of "detection bias" in epidemiologic rates of disease. *Transactions of the Association of American Physicians, 87*, 180–185.

Feldman, J., & Eysenck, S.B.G. (1986). Addictive personality traits in bulimic patients. *Personality & Individual Differences, 7*, 923–926.

Fisher, R.A. (1959). *Smoking: The cancer controversy.* Edinburgh: Oliver & Boyd.

Fleiss, J.L. (1987). *Statistical methods for rates and proportions.* New York: Wiley.

Fox, B.H. (1978). Premorbid psychological factors as related to incidence of cancer. *Journal of Behavioural Medicine, 1*, 45–133.

Fox, B.H. (1981a). Behavioral issues in cancer. in S.M. Weiss, J.A. Herd, & B.H. Fox (Eds.), *Perspectives on behavioral medicine* (pp. 101–134). London: Academic Press.

Fox, B.H. (1981b). Psychosocial factors and the immune system in human cases. In R. Ader (Ed.), *Psychoneuroimmunology* (pp. 103–158). Orlando, FL: Academic Press.

Fox, B.H. (1983) Current theory of psychogenic effects on cancer incidence and prognosis. *Journal of Psychosocial Oncology, 1*, 17–31.

Fox, B.H., & Temoshok, L. (1988). Mind–body and behavior in cancer incidence. *Advances, Institute for the Advancement of Health, 5*, 41–56.

Friedman, A.F., Webb, J.TT., & Lewak, R. (1989). *Psychological assessment with the MMPI.* London: Lawrence Erlbaum.

Friedman, G.D., Siegelaub, A.B., Dales, L.G., & Seltzer, C.C. (1979). Characteristic predictions of coronary heart disease in ex-smokers before they stopped smoking: Comparisons with persistent smokers and non-smokers. *Journal of Chronic Diseases, 32*, 175–190.

Friedman, H.S., & Booth-Kewley, S. (1987). The "disease-prone personality." *American Psychologist, 42*, 534–555.

Friedman, M. (1987). Effect of modifying Type A behavior after myocardial infarction in recurrence rates. *Mount Sinai Journal of Medicine*, *51*, 47–55.

Friedman, M., Thorensen, C., Gill, J., Powell, L., Ulmer, D., Thompson, l., Price, V., Rabin, D., Breall, W., Dixon, T., Levy, R., & Bourg, E. (1984). Alterations of type A behavior and reduction in cardiac recurrence in postmyocardial infarction patients. *American Heart Journal*, *108*, 237–248.

Friedman, M., Thorensen, C.E., Gill, J.J., Ulmer, D., Powell, L.H., Price, V.A., Brown, B., Thompson, L., Rabin, D.D., Breall, W.S., Bourg, E., Levy, R., & Dixon, T. (1986). Alteration of type A behaviour and its effect of cardiac recurrences in postmyocardial infarction patients: Summary results of the recurrent coronary heart prevention project. *American Heart Journal*, *112*, 653–665.

Fries, J., Green, L., & Levine, S. (1985). Health promotions and the comparison of morbidity. *Lancet*, March 4, 481–483.

Frith, C.D. (1971). Smoking behavior and its relation to smokers' immediate experience. *British Journal of Social Psychology*, *10*, 73–78.

Galtung, J. (1967). *Theory and methods of social research*. London: Allen and Unwin.

Gao, Y., Blot, W., Zheng, W., Franmini, J. & Hsu, L. (1988). Lung cancer and smoking in Shanghai. *International Journal of Epidemiology*, *17*, 277–280.

Gill, J.J., Price, V.A. Friedman, M., Thorensen, L.E., Powell, L.N., Ulmer, D., Brown, B., & Drews, F.R. (1985). Reduction in type A behavior in healthy middle-aged American military officers. *American Heart Journal*, *110*, 503–514.

Glaser, R., & Kiecolt-Glaser, J. (1985). "Relatively mild stress" depresses cellular immunity in healthy adults. *Behavior & Brain Science*, *8*, 401–403.

Glaser, R., Kiecolt-Glaser, J., Speicher, C., & Holliday, J. (1985). Stress, loneliness and changes in herpes virus latency. *Journal of Behavioral Medicine*, *8*, 249–260.

Glaser, R., Kiecolt-Glaser, J., Start, J.C., Tarr, K.L., Speicher, C.E., & Halliday, J. (1986). Stress-related impairments in cellular immunity. *Psychiatric Research*, *16*, 233–239.

Glaser, R., Thorn, B.E., Tarr, K.L., Kiecolt-Glaser, J., & D'Ambrosia, S. (1985). Effects of stress on methyltransferase synthesis: An important DNA repair enzyme. *Health Psychology*, *4*, 403–412.

Gordon, T., Kannel, W., & McGee, D. (1974). Death and coronary heart attacks in men after giving up cigarette smoking. A report from the Framingham Study. *Lancet*, *7*, 1345–1348.

Gossop, M.R. (Ed.) (1989). *Relapse and addictive behaviour*. London: Routledge.

Gossop, M.R., & Eysenck, S.B.G. (1980). A further investigation into the personality of drug addicts in treatment. *British Journal of Addiction*, *75*, 305–311.

Green, J.P., & Art, P.B. (1982). Carcinoma of the lung in non-smoking Chinese women. *Western Journal of Medicine*, *136*, 291–294.

Green, R.G., & Green, M.L. (1987). Relaxation increases salivary immunoglobin A[1]. *Psychological Reports*, *61*, 623–629.

Greer, S., Morris, T., & Pettingale, K.W. (1979). Psychological response to cancer: Effect on outcome. *Lancet*, *2*, 785–787.

Grizzle, J.E., Starmer, C.E., & Koch, G.G. (1969). Analysis of categorical data by linear models. *Biometrics*, *25*, 489–504.

Grossarth-Maticek, R. (1980a). Social psychotherapy and course of the disease. *Psychotherapy and Psychosomatics*, *33*, 129–138.

Grossarth-Maticek, R. (1980b). Synergistic effects of cigarette smoking, systolic blood pressure and psychosocial risk factors for lung cancer, cardiac infact and Apoplexy Cerebri. *Psychotherapy and Psychosomatics*, *34*, 267–272.

Grossarth-Maticek, R. (1986). Psychosociale Verhaltenstypen und chronische Erkrankungen. *Der Kassenarzt*, *39*, 26–35.

Grossarth-Maticek, R. (1989). Disposition, Exposition, Verhaltensmuster, Organsverschädigung und Stimulierung des Zentralen Nervensystems in der Ätiologie des Brochial-, Magen-, und Leber Karzinoma. *Deutsche Zeitschrift für Onkologie*, *21*, 62–78.

Grossarth-Maticek, R., Bastiaans, J., & Kanazir, D.T. (1985). Psychosocial factors as strong predictors of mortality from cancer, ischaemic heart disease and stroke: The Yugoslav prospective study. *Journal of Psychosomatic Research*, *29*, 167–176.

Grossarth-Maticek, R., & Eysenck, H.J. (1989a). Is media information that smoking causes illness a self-fulfilling prophecy? *Psychological Reports*, *65*, 177–178.

Grossarth-Maticek, R., & Eysenck, H.J. (1989b). Length of survival and lymphocyte percentage in women with mammary cancer as a function of psychotherapy. *Psychological Reports*, *65*, 315–321.

Grossarth-Maticek, R., & Eysenck, H.J. (1990). Prophylactic effects of psychoanalysis on cancer-prone and coronary heart disease-prone probands, as compared with control groups and behavior therapy groups. *Journal of Behavior Therapy and Experimental Psychiatry*, *21*, 91–99.

Grossarth-Maticek, R., & Eysenck, H.J. (1991). Creative novation behaviour therapy as a prophylactic treatment for cancer and coronary heart disease: I. Description of treatment. *Behavioral Research and Therapy*. *29*, 1–16

Grossarth-Maticek, R., & Eysenck, H.J. (in press-a). Personality and stress as synergistic risk factors for cancer and coronary heart disease, in interaction with smoking, genetic predisposition, and chronic bronchitis. *Integrative Physiological and Behavioral Science*.

Grossarth-Maticek, R., & Eysenck, H.J. (in press-b). An improved method for obtaining accurate estimates of consumption rates. *Psychological Reports*.

Grossarth-Maticek, R., Eysenck, H.J., Gallasch, B., Vetter, H., & Frentzel-Beyme, R. (in press). Changes in degree of sclerosis as a function of prophylactic treatment in cancer-prone and CHD-prone probands. *Behaviour Research and Therapy*.

Grossarth-Maticek, R., Eysenck, H.J., Uhlenbruck, G., Rieder, H., Vetter, H., Freeseman, C., Rakic, L., Gallasch, G., Kanazir, D.T., & Liesen, H. (1990). Sport activity and personality as elements in preventing cancer and coronary heart disease. *Perceptual and Motor Skills*, *71*, 199–209.

Grossarth-Maticek, R., Eysenck, H.J., & Vetter, H. (1988). Personality type, smoking habit and their interaction as predictors of cancer and coronary heart disease. *Personality & Individual Differences*, *9*, 479–495.

Grossarth-Maticek, R., Eysenck, H.J., Vetter, H., & Schmidt, P. (1988). Psychosocial types and chronic diseases: Results of the Heidelberg Prospective Psychosomatic Intervention Study. In S. Maes, C. Spielberger, P, Defares, & I.G. Sarason (Eds.), *Topics in health psychology* (pp. 57–75). London: John Wiley & Sons.

Grossarth-Maticek, R., Kanazir, D.T., Schmidt, P., & Vetter, H. (1982). Psychosomatic factors in the process of cancerogenesis. *Psychotherapy and Psychosomatics, 28*, 284–302.

Grossarth-Maticek, R., Kanazir, D.T., Vetter, H., & Jankovic, M. (1983). Smoking as a risk factor for lung cancer and cardiac infarct as mediated by psychosocial variables. *Psychotherapy and Psychosomatics, 39*, 94–105.

Grossarth-Maticek, R., Schmidt, P., Vetter, H., & Arndt, S. (1984). Psychotherapy research in oncology. In A. Steptoe & A. Mathews (Eds.), *Health care and human behaviour* (pp. 325–341). London: Academic Press.

Grossarth-Maticek, R., Siegrist, J., & Vetter, H. (1982). Interpersonal regression as a predictor of cancer. *Social Science and Medicine, 16*, 493–498.

Grossarth-Maticek, R., Vetter, H., & Frentzel-Beyme, R. (1988). Precursor lesions of the GI tract and psychosocial risk factors for prediction and prevention of gastric cancer. *Cancer Detection and Prevention, 13*, 23–29.

Grundmann, E., Clemmesen, J., & Muir, C.S. (Eds.). (1982). *Geographical pathology in cancer epidemiology*. New York: G. Fischer Verlag.

Gruver, R.H., & Freis, E.D. (1957). A study of diagnostic error. *Annals of Internal Medicine, 47*, 108–120.

Guberan, E. (1979). Surprising decline of cardiovascular mortality in Switzerland: 1951–1976. *Journal of Epidemiology and Community Health, 33*, 114–120.

Gunning-Schepers, L., Barrendregt, R., & Maas, J. (1989). Population interventions reassessed. *Lancet, 1*, 479–481.

Hager, E.D. (Ed.). (1986). *Biomodulation und Biotherapie des Krebses*. Heidelberg, Germany: E. Fischer.

Hammond, E.C. (1966). Smoking in relation to death rates of one million men and women. *National Cancer Institute Monographs, 19*, 122–204.

Hanson, P. (1987). *The joy of stress*. London: Pan.

Hartveit, F. (1979). Autopsy findings in cases with a clinically uncertain diagnosis. *Journal of Pathology, 129*, 111–119.

Harvald, B., Hauge, M. (1963). Hereditary factors elucidated by twin studies. In J.V. Weel, M.V. Shaw, & W.J. Schull (Eds.), *Genetics and the epidemiology of chronic diseases*. Washington, DC: Public Health Service.

Heasman, M.A., & Lipworth, L. (1966). *Accuracy of certification of cause of death*. London: H.M.S.O.

Heller, W.-D. (1983). Lung cancer and passive smoking. *Lancet, 2*, 1309.

Hinds. M., Stemmermann, G., Yang, H., Kolome, L., Lee, J. & Wegner, E. (1981). Differences in lung cancer risk from smoking among Japanese, Chinese and Hawaiian women in Hawaii. *International Journal of Cancer, 27*, 297–302.

Hirayama, T. (1981a). Non-smoking wives of heavy smokers have a higher risk of lung cancer: A study from Japan. *British Medical Journal, 1*, 183–185.

Hirayama, T. (1981b). Non-smoking wives of heavy smokers have a higher risk of lung cancer: A study from Japan. *British Medical Journal, 2*, 916–917.

Hirayama, T. (1981c). Non-smoking wives of heavy smokers have a higher risk of lung cancer: A study from Japan. *British Medical Journal, 2*, 1466.

Holme, I. (1982). On the separation of intervention effects of diet and antismoking advice on the incidence of major coronary events in coronary high risk men. The Oslo Study. *Journal of the Oslo City Hospital, 32*, 31–54.

Holmes, T.H., & Rahe, R.H. (1967). The social readjustment rating scale. *Journal of Psychosomatic Research, 11*, 213–218.

Hopkins, P.N., & Williams, R.R. (1981). A survey of 246 suggested coronary risk factors. *Atherosclerosis, 40*, 1–52.

Hutchinson, G.B. (1968). The nature of epidemiologic evidence: smoking and health. *Bulletin of the New York Academy of Medicine, 44*, 1471–1475.

Hypertension-Detection and Follow-up Program Co-operative Group. (1988). Persistence of reduction in blood pressure and mortality of participants in the Hypertension Detection and Follow-up Program. *Journal of American Medical Association, 259*, 2113–2122.

Irwin, M., Daniels, E.T., Bloom, T.L., Smith, H., & Weiner, H. (1987). Life events, depressive symptoms, and immune function. *American Journal of Psychiatry, 144*, 437–441.

Irwin, M., Vale, W., & Britton, K. (1987). Central cortico-tropin-releasing factor suppressor natural killer cell cytotoxicity. *Brain, Behavior and Immunity, 1*, 81–87.

Janerich, D.T., Thompson, W.D., Varela, L.R., Greenwald, P., Chorost, S., Tucci, C., Zaman, M.B., Melamed, M.R., Kiely, M., & McKneally, M.F. (1990). Lung cancer and exposure to tobacco smoke in the household. *The New England Journal of Medicine*, Sept. 6, 632–636.

Jarvis, M., West, R., Tunstall-Pedoe, H., & Vesey, C. (1984). An evaluation of the intervention against smoking with Multiple Risk Factor Intervention Trial. *Preventive Medicine, 13*, 501–509.

Jemmott, J.B. (1987). Social motives and susceptibility to disease: Stalking individual differences in health risks. *Journal of Personality, 55*, 267–298.

Jemmott, J.B., & Locke, S.E. (1984). Psychosocial factors, immunologic mediation, and human susceptibility to infectious diseases: How much do we know? *Psychological Bulletin, 95*, 78–108.

Jemmott, J.B., & Magloire, K. (1988). Academic stress, social support, and secretory immunoglobin A. *Journal of Personality & Social Psychology, 55*, 803–810.

Johnston, D.W. (1989). Will stress management prevent coronary heart disease? *The Psychologist, 2*, 275–278.

Justice, A. (1985). Review of the effects of stress on cancer in laboratory animals: Importance of time of stress application and type of tumor. *Psychological Bulletin, 98*, 108–138.

Kagan, A., Katsuki, S., Sternley, N., & Vanecek, R. (1967). Reliability of death certificate data on vascular lesions affecting the central nervous system. *Bulletin of The World Health Organization, 37*, 477–483.

Kahn, M.A. (1966). The Dorn study of smoking and mortality among U.S. veterans: Report on eight and one-half years of observation. *National Cancer Institute Monographs, 19*, 1–125.

Kanazir, D.T., Djordjevic-Markovic, R., & Grossarth-Maticek, R. (1984). Psychosocial (emotional) stress, steroid hormones, and carcinogenesis: Molecular aspects. In Y.A. Evchinnikov (Ed.), *Progress in bioorganic chemistry and molecular biology* (pp. 509–520). Amsterdam, The Netherlands: Elsevier.

Kannel, W.B. (1981). Update on the role of cigarette smoking in coronary heart disease. *American Health Journal, 101*, 319–327.

Kannel, W.B., D'Agostino, R.B., & Belanger, A.J. (1987). Fibrinogen, cigarette smoking and risk of cardiovascular disease: Insights from the Framingham Study. *American Heart Journal, 113*, 1006–1010.

Kannel, W.B., & Gordon, T. (1970). *The Framingham study. An epidemiological investigation of cardiovascular disease.* Washington, DC: National Institutes of Health.

Kannel, W.B., Neaton, J.D., and Wentworth, D. (1986). Overall and coronary heart disease mortality rates in relation to major risk factors in 325,348 men screened for the MRFIT. *American Heart Journal, 112,* 825–836.

Kaplan, J.R., Manuck, S.B., Clarkson, T.B., Lusso, F.M., Taub, D.M., & Miller, E.W. (1978). Social stress and atherosclerosis in normocholesterolemic monkeys. *Science, 220,* 733–735.

Katz, L. (1969). *Hearings on cigarette labelling and advertising: 2.* Washington, DC: Committee on Interstate and Foreign Commerce, House of Representatives.

Kennedy, S., Kiecolt-Glaser, J., & Glaser, R. (1988). Immunological consequences of acute and chronic stressors: Mediating role of interpersonal relationships. *British Journal of Medical Psychology, 61,* 77–85.

Kern, W.H., Jones, J.C., & Chapman, V.D. (1968). Pathology of bronchogenic carcinoma in long term survivors. *Cancer, 21,* 772–780.

Keys, A. (1962). Diet and coronary heart disease throughout the world. *Cardiological Practice, 13,* 225–244.

Kiecolt-Glaser, J., Garner, W., Speicher, C., Penn, G., Halliday, J., & Glaser, R. (1984). Psychosocial modifiers of immunocompetence in medical students. *Psychosomatic Medicine, 46,* 7–14.

Kiecolt-Glaser, J., Glaser, R., Williger, D., Stunt, J., Merrick, G., Sheppard, S., Rickers, D., Romisker, C., Briner, W., Bonnell, G., & Domenberg, R. (1985). Psychological enhancement of immunocompetence in a geriatric population. *Health Psychology,* 25–41.

Kiecolt-Galser, J., Rickers, D., George, J., Merrick, G., Speicher, C.E., Garner, W., & Glaser, R. (1984). Unitary corticol levels, cellular incompetency, and loneliness in psychiatric inpatients. *Psychosomatic Medicine, 46,* 15–23.

Kleinbaum, D.G., Kupper, L.L., & Morganstern, H. (1982). *Epidemiological research: Principles and quantitative methods* Belmont, CA: Lifetime Learning Publications. (pp. 403–418).

Knorring, L. von, & Oreland, L. (1985). Personality traits and platelet monoamine oxidase in tobacco smokers. *Psychological Medicine, 15,* 327–334.

Kooperman, J.S. (1981). Interaction between discrete causes. *American Journal of Epidemiology, 113,* 716–724.

Korneva, E.A., Klimenko, V.M., & Shkhinek, E.K. (1985). *Neurohormonal maintenance of immune homeostasis.* Chicago: The University of Chicago Press.

Kune, G.A., Kunc, S., Watson, L.F., & Bahnson, C.B. (in press). Personality as a risk factor in large bowel cancer. *Psychological Medicine.*

Laudenslager, M.L., Ryan, S.M., Drugan, R.C., Hyson, R.C., & Maier, S.F. (1983). Coping and immunosuppression: Inseparable but not escapable stock suppresses lymphocyte proliferation. *Science, 221,* 568–570.

Leaventon, P.E., Barlie, P.D., Kleinman, J.C., Dannenberg, S.L., Kannel, W.B., & Carnun-Hambley, J.C. (1987). Representativeness of the Framingham Risk Model for coronary heart disease mortality: a comparison with a national cohort study. *Journal of Chronic Diseases, 40,* 775–784.

Lee, P.N. (1981). Non-smoking wives of heavy smokers have a higher risk of lung cancer: a study from Japan. *British Medical Journal, 2,* 1465–1466.

Le Fanu, J. (1987). *Eat your heart out: The fallacy of the "healthy diet"*. London: Macmillan.

Leren, P., Askevold, O., Froiti, A., Grymyr, D., Helgeland, A., Hjermann, I., Holme, I., Lund-Larsen, P., & Norum, K. (1975). The Oslo study. Cardiovascular disease in middle-aged and young Oslo men. *Acta Medica Scandinavica [Supplement]*, *5888*, 1–38.

Leung, J. (1977). Cigarette smoking, the kerosene stove and lung cancer in Hong Kong. *British Journal of Distance Chest*, *71*, 273–276.

Levy, S. (1985). *Behaviour and cancer*. London: Jossey-Bass.

Levy, S., Herberman, R., Lippman, M., & d'Angelo, T. (1987). Correlation of stess factors with sustained depression of natural killer cell activity and predicted prognosis in patients with breast cancer. *Journal Clinical Oncology*, *5*, 348–353.

Levy, S., Herberman, R.B., Maluish, A.M., Schlien, B., & Lippman, M. (1985). Prospective risk assessment in primary breast cancer: Behavioural and immunological parameters. *Health Psychology*, *4*, 99–113.

Linn, B.S., Linn, M.W., & Jensen, J. (1981). Anxiety and immune repressiveness. *Psychological Reports*, *49*, 969–970.

Linn, M.W., Linn, B.S., & Jensen, J. (1984). Stressful events, dysphoric mood, and immune responsiveness. *Psychological Reports*, *54*, 219–222.

Linn, B., Linn, M., & Klimas, N. (1988). Effects of psychophysical stress on surgical outcome. *Psychosomatic Medicine*, *50*, 230–244.

Lovibond, S.H., Birrell, P.C., & Langeluddecke, P. (1986). Changing coronary heart disease risk-factor states: The effects of three behavioural programs. *Journal of Behavioral Medicine*, *9*, 915–937.

Lyon, J.L., Gardner, J.W., & West, D.W. (1980). Cancer incidence in Mormons and non-Mormons in Utah during 1967–75. *Journal of the National Cancer Institute*, *65*, 1063–1071.

MacMahon, S. (1987). Alcohol consumption and hypertension. *Hypertension*, *9*, 111–121.

MacMahon, S., Peto, R., Cutler, J., Collins, R., Gorlie, P., Matan, H., Abbot, R., Godwin, J., Dyer, A., & Stamler, J. (1990). Blood pressure, stroke, and coronary heart disease. *Lancet*, *335*, 765–774.

Mainland, D., & Herrera, L. (1956). The risk of biased selection in forward going surveys with non-professional interviewers. *Journal of Chronic Diseases*, *4*, 240–244.

Mann, G.V. (1977). Diet-heart: End of an era. *The New England Journal of Medicine*, Sept. 22, 644–649.

Mantel, N. (1981). Non-smoking wives of heavy smokers have a higher risk of lung cancer: A study from Japan. *British Medical Journal*, *2*, 914–915.

Mantel, N., & Haenszel, W. (1959). Statistical aspects of the analysis of data from retrospective studies of disease. *Journal of the National Cancer Institute*, *22*, 789–798.

McCarthy, E.G. & Widmer, G.W. (1974). Effects of screening by consultants on recommended elective surgical procedures. *The New England Journal of Medicine*, *291*, 1331–1335.

McClelland, D.C. (1989). Motivational factors in health and disease. *American Psychology*, *44*, 675–683.

McCleeland, D.C., Floor, E., Davidson, R.J., & Saron, C. (1980). Stressed power motivation, sympathetic activation, immune function and illness. *Journal of Human Stress*, *6*, 11–19.

McCleeland, D.C., Ross, G., & Patel, V. (1985). The effects of an academic examination on salivary norepinephrine and immunoglobin levels. *Journal of Human Stress, 11,* 52–59.

McCormick, J., & Skrabanek, P. (1988). Coronary heart disease is not preventable by population interventions. *Lancet, 2,* 839–841.

McLennan, R., da Costa, J., Day, N.E., Law, C.H., Ng, Y.K., & Shanmugaratnam, K. (1977). Risk factors for lung cancer in Singapore Chinese, a population with high female incidence rates. *International Journal of Cancer, 20,* 854–860.

McMichael, A.J. (1978). Increases in laryngeal cancer in Britain and Australia in relation to alcohol and tobacco consumption trends. *Lancet,* June 10, 1244–1247.

McMichael, J. (1979). Fats and atheroma: An inquest. *British Medical Journal,* Jan. 20, 173–175.

Medical charities and prevention. (1971). [Editorial.] *British Medical Journal, 2,* 1616.

Meehl, P.E. (1990). Why summaries of research on psychological theories are often uninterpretable [Monograph]. *Psychological Reports, 1,* (Suppl. 1).

Miettinen, T.A., Huttunen, J., Naukkarinen, V., Strandberg, T., Mattila, S., Kumlin, T., & Saura, S. (1985). Multifactorial primary prevention of cardiovascular diseases in middle-aged men: Risk-factor changes, incidence and mortality. *Journal of the American Medical Association, 254,* 2097–2101.

Miller, N. (1983). Behavioral Medicine: Symbiosis between laboratory and clinic. *American Review of Psychology, 34,* 1–31.

Miller, N. (1985). Effects of emotional stress in the immune system. *Pavlovian Journal of Biological Science, 20,* 47–52.

Miller, S.M. (1981). Predictability and human stress: Toward a clarification of evidence and theory. *Advances in Experimental Social Psychology, 14,* 203–256.

Monjem, A.A. (1984). Effects of acute and chronic stress upon lymphocyte blastogenesis in mice and humans. In E.L. Cooper (Ed.), *Stress, immunity, and aging* (pp. 81–108). New York: Marcel Dekker.

Muldoon, M.E., Manuck, S.B., & Matthews, K.A. (1990). Lowering cholesterol concentrations and mortality: a qualitative review of primary prevention trials. *British Medical Journal, 301,* 309–314.

Multiple Risk Factor Intervention Trial Research Group. (1982). Multiple risk factor intervention trial. *Journal of the American Medical Association, 248,* 1465–1477.

Multiple Risk Factor Intervention Trial Research Group. (1990). Mortality rates after 10–15 years for participants in the Multiple Risk Factor Intervention Trial. *Journal of the American Medical Association, 263,* 1795–1801.

Murphy, J.A., Monson, R.P., Sobol, A.M., & Leighton, A.H. (1987). Affiliated disorders and mortality. *Archives of General Psychiatry, 44,* 473–480.

National Health and Medical Research Council. (1987). *Effects of passive smoking on health.* Canberra, Australia: Australian Government Publicity Service.

Nelson, D.V., Friedman, L.C., Baer, P.E., Lane, M., & Smith, F.E. (1989). Attitudes to cancer: Psychometric properties of fighting spirit and denial. *Journal of Behavioral Medicine, 12,* 341–355.

Nemeroff, C., Widerloo, E., Bissette, G., Walleus, H., Karlsson, I., Eklund, R., Kilts, C., Larsen, P., & Vale, W. (1984). Elevated concentrations of cortico-tropin-releasing factor-like activity in depressed patients. *Science*, *226*, 1342–1344.

O'Connor, K., & Stravynski, A. (1982). Evaluation of a smoking typology by use of a specific behavioral substitution method of self-control. *Behaviour Research and Therapy*, *20*, 279–288.

Oeser, H. (1979). *Krebs: Schicksal oder Verschuldung?* Stuttgart: Thieme.

Oliver, M.F. (1982). Does control of risk factors prevent coronary heart disease? *British Medical Journal*, *285*, 1065–1066.

Oliver, M.F. (1988). Reducing cholesterol does not reduce mortality. *Journal of the American College of Cardiology*, *12*, 814–817.

Otis, M.A. (1924). A study of suggestibility in children. *Archives of Psychology*, *11*(70).

Paganini-Hill, A., Char, A., Ross, R.K., & Henderson, B.E. (1989). Aspirin use and chronic disease: A cohort study of the elderly. *British Medical Journal*, *299*, 1247–1250.

Passey, R.D. (1961). Some problems of lung cancer. *Lancet*, *2*, 107–112.

Patel, C., Marmot, M.G.B., Terry, D.J., Carruthers, M., Hunt, B., & Patel, M. (1985). Trial of relaxation in reducing coronary risk: Four year follow-up. *British Medical Journal*, *290*, 1103–1186.

Pearl, R. (1925). *The rate of living*. New York: Knopf.

Pennebaker, J.W. (1985). Traumatic experience and psychosomatic disease: Exploring the roles of behavioral inhibition, obsession, and confiding. *Canadian Psychology*, *26*, 82–95.

Pennebaker, J.W. (1989). Confession, inhibition and disease. In L. Berkowitz (Ed.), *Advances in experimental social psychology* (Vol. 22, pp. 211–244). Orlando, FL: Academic Press.

Pennebaker, J.W., Kiecolt-Glaser, J., & Glaser, R. (1988). Disclosure of traumas and immune function: Health implications for psychotherapy. *Journal of Consulting and Clinical Psychology*, *56*, 235–245.

Perkins, D.A. (1989). Interaction among coronary heart disease risk factors. *Annals of Behavioral Medicine*, *11*, 3–11.

Perkins, K.A. (1985). The synergistic effect of smoking and serum cholesterol on coronary heart disease. *Health Psychology*, *4*, 337–360.

Perkins, K.A., (1987). Use of terms to describe results: "Additive," "synergistic." *Psychophysiology*, *24*, 719–720.

Pettingale, K.W., Morris, T., Greer, S., & Haybittle, J.L. (1985). Mental attitudes to cancer: An additional, prognostic factor. *Lancet*, *2*, 750.

Pettingale, K.W., Philalithis, A., Tee, D., & Greer, H.S. (1981). The biological correlates of psychological responses to breast cancer. *Journal of Psychosomatic Research*, *25*, 453–458.

Physicians' Health Study Research Group. Preliminary report: Findings from the aspirin component of the ongoing Physicians' Health Study. *New England Journal of Medicine*, *318*, 262–264.

Pike, M.C., & Doll, R. (1965). Age at onset of lung cancer: Significance in relation to effect of smoking. *Lancet*, *1*, 665–668.

Plackett, R.L. (1974). *The analysis of categorical data*. London: Griffin.

Ploeg, H. van der, Kleijn, W.C., Mook, J., Hunge, M. van, Pieters, A., & Leer, J-W. (1989). Rationality and antiemotionality as a risk factor for cancer: Concept differentiation. *Journal of Psychosomatic Research*, *33*, 217–225.

Plomin, R., & Bergeman, C.S. (in press). The nature of nurture: Genetic influence on "environmental" measures. *Behavioral and Brain Sciences*.

Plotnikoff, N., Faith, R., Murgo, A., & Good, R.A. (Eds.). (1986). *Enkephalines and endorphins: Stress and the immune system*. New York: Plenum Press.

Pohler, G. (1989). *Krebs und Seelischer Konflikt*. Frankfurt, Germany: Nexus.

Pomerleau, V.E., & Pomerleau, C.S. (1984). Neuroregulators and the reinforcement of smoking: Towards a biobehavioral explanation. *Neuroscience and Biobehavioral Reviews, 8*, 503–513.

Price, V.A. (1982). *Type A behavior pattern*. New York: Academic Press.

Puska, P., Tuomilehito, J., & Saloney, J. (1979). Changes in coronary risk factors during a comprehensive five-year community programme to control cardio-vascular disease. *British Medical Journal, 2*, 1173–1178.

Rigdon, R.H., & Kirchoff, H. (1953). Smoking and cancer of the lung—Let's review the facts. *Texas Reports on Biology and Medicine, 11*, 715–727.

Quander-Blaznik, J. (1991). Personality as a predictor of lung cancer: A replication. *Personality Individual Differences, 12*, 125–130.

Reid, D.D., & Rose, G.A. (1964). Assessing the comparability of mortality statistics. *British Medical Journal, 2*, 1437–1439.

Roberts, J.L., & Graveling, P.A. (1986). *The big kill*. Health Education Council and the British Medical Association for N.W. London: Regional Health Authority.

Rodin, J. (1984). Managing the stress of aging: The role of control and coping. In S. Levine, & H. Urrin (Eds.), *Coping and Health* (pp. 171–202). New York: Plenum.

Rodin, J. (1986). Health, control and aging. In M. Baltes & P.B. Baltes (Eds.), *Aging and the psychology of control* (pp. 83–92). Hillsdale, NJ: Lawrence Erlbaum.

Roos, B., Vernet, J., & Abelin, T. (Eds.). (1989). *Rauchen und Sterblichkeit in der Schweiz*. Bern; Bundesamt für Gesundheitswesen.

Rose, G., & Hamilton, P.J.S. (1978). A randomized controlled trial of the effect on middle-aged men of advice to stop smoking. *Journal of Epidemiology and Community Health, 32*, 275–281.

Rose, G., Hamilton, P., Colvell, L., & Shipley, M. (1982). A randomized controlled trial of anti-smoking advice: 10-year results. *Journal of Epidemiology and Community Health, 36*, 102–108.

Rosenblatt, M.B. (1974). Lung cancer and smoking—The evidence reassessed. *New Science*, May, 332.

Rosenblatt, M.B., Teng, P.K., Kerpe, S., & Beck, I. (1971). Prevalence of lung cancer: Disparity between clinical and autopsy certification. *Medical Counterpoint, 33*, 53–59.

Rosenman, R.H., & Chesney, M.A. (1980). The relationship of type of behaviour to coronary heart disease. *Activas Nervosa Superior, 22*, 1–45.

Rothman, K.J. (1974). Synergy and antagonism in cause–effect relationships. *American Journal of Epidemiology, 99*, 385–388.

Rothman, K.J., & Keller, A.Z. (1972). The effect of joint exposure to alcohol and tobacco on risk of cancer of the mouth and pharynx. *Journal of Chronic Disease, 23*, 711–716.

Rothman, K.J., Cann, C.I., Flanders, D., & Fried, M.P. (1980). Epidemiology of laryngeal cancer. *Epidemiology Review, 2*, 195–209.

Rou, B., Rose, J., Sunderland, T., Moritisa, J., & Murphy, D. (1988). Antisomatostatin G in major depressive disorder. A preliminary study with implications for autoimmune mechanisms of depression. *Archives of General Psychiatry, 45*, 924–928.

Royal College of Physicians. (1971). *Smoking and health now.* London: Pitman.

Saracci, R. (1987). The interactions of tobacco smoking and other agents in cancer etiology. *Epidemiology Review, 9*, 135–193.

Saracci, R., & Riboli, E. (1989). Passive smoking and lung cancer: Current evidence and ongoing research at the International Agency for Research and Cancer. *Mutation Research, 222*, 117–127.

Schatzkin, A., Hoover, R.N., Taylor, P.R., Ziegler, R.C., Carter, C.L., Albans, D., Larson, D.B., & Licitra, L.M. (1988). Site-specific analysis of total serum cholesterol and incident cancer in the National Health and Nutrition Examination Survey: 1. Epidemiologic follow-up study. *Cancer Research, 48*, 452–458.

Scheier, M.F., Matthews, K.A., Owens, J.F., Magorem, G.J., Lefevre, R.C., Abbot, R.A., & Carver, C.S. (1989). Dispositional optimism and recovery from coronary artery bypass surgery: The beneficial effects of physical and psychosocial well-being. *Journal of Personality and Social Psychology, 57*, 1024–1040.

Schleifer, S., Keller, S., Meyerson, A., Roskin, M., Davis, K., & Stein, M. (1984). Lymphocyte function in major depressive disorders. *Archives of General Psychiatry, 41*, 484–486.

Schmale, A.H., & Iker, H. (1971). Hopelessness as a predictor of cervical cancer. *Social Science and Medicine, 5*, 95–100.

Schmitz, P. (1990, July). *Personality, stress and psychosomatics.* Paper presented at the Fifth European Conference on Personality, Ariccia, Italy.

Sehrt, E. (1904). *Beiträge zur Kenntnis des Primären Lungencarcinoma.* Leipzig, Germany: George.

Seligman, M.E.P. (1975). *Helplessness.* San Francisco: W.H. Freeman.

Seltzer, C.C. (1968). An evaluation of the effect of smoking on coronary heart disease. *Journal of the American Medical Association, 203*, 193–200.

Seltzer, C.C. (1989). Framingham study data and "established wisdom" about cigarette smoking and coronary heart disease. *Journal of Clinical Epidemiology, 42*, 743–750.

Shavit, Y., Lewis, J., Terman, G., Gale, R., & Leibeskind, J. (1989). Opioid peptides mediate the suppressive effects of stress on natural killer cell cytotoxicity. *Science, 223*, 188–190.

Simarak, S., de Jong, U.W., Breslow, N., Dahl, C.J., Ruckphaopunt, K., Scheelings, P., & MacLennan, R. (1977). Cancer of the oral cavity, pharynx/ larynx and lung in North Thailand: Case control study and analysis of cigar smoke. *British Journal of Cancer, 36*, 130–140.

Smithers, D.W. (1935). Facts and fancies about cancer of the lung. *British Medical Journal, 1*, 1235–1239.

Solomon, G. (1985). The emerging field of psychoneuroimmunology. *Advances, 2*, 6–19.

Solomon, G. (1987). Psychoneuroimmunology: Interaction between central nervous system and immune system. *Journal of Neuroscience Research, 18*, 1–9.

Solomon, G., Levine, S., & Kraft, J. (1968). Early experience and immunity. *Nature*, *220*, 821–822.

Solomon, G., & Moos, R. (1964). Emotions, immunity and disease: A speculative theoretical intergration. *Archives of General Psychiatry*, *11*, 657–674.

Solvason, H., Ghanta, V., & Hiramoto, R. (1988). Conditional augmentation of natural killer cell activity. Independence of interferon-beta. *Journal of Immunology*, *140*, 661–665.

Spiegel, D., Bloom, J.R., Kraemer, H.C., & Gottleib, E. (1989). Effect of psychosocial treatment on survival of patients with metastatic breast cancer. *Lancet*, *2*, 888–891.

Spielberger, C.D. (1986). Psychological determinants of smoking behavior. In R.D. Tollison (Ed.), *Smoking and society* (pp. 89–134). Toronto: Lexington Books.

Stebbings, J.H. (1971). Chronic respiratory disease among non-smokers in Hagerstown, Maryland: 2. Problems in the estimation of pulmonary function values in epidemiological surveys. *Environmental Research*, *4*, 163–192.

Stell, P.M. (1972). Smoking and laryngeal cancer. *Lancet*, *1*, 617–618.

Steptoe, A. (1981). *Psychological factors in cardiovascular disorders*. New York: Academic Press.

Steptoe, A. (1989). Coping and psychophysiological reaction. In S. Miller (Ed.). *Advances in Behaviour Research and Therapy*, [Special Issue], *11* (4), 259–270.

Sterling, T.D. (1973). The statistician vis-à-vis issues of public health. *The American Statistician*, *27*, 212–217.

Sterling, T.D. (1977). New evidence concerning smoking and health. *Medical Journal of Australia*, Oct. 15, 538–542.

Stolley, P.D. (in press). When genius errs: R.A. Fischer and the lung cancer controversy. *American Journal of Epidemiology*.

Stone, A.A., Cox, D.S., Valdimarsdottir, H., Jandorf, L., & Neale, J.G. (1987). Evidence that secretory IgA antibody is associated with daily mood. *Journal of Personality and Social Psychology*, *52*, 988–993.

Taylor, S.E. (1990). Health pychology. *American Psychology*, *45*, 40–50.

Temoshok, L. (1985). Biopsychological studies on cutaneous malignant melanoma: Psychological factors associated with prognostic indicators, progression, psychophysiology, and tumour-host response. *Social Science and Medicine*, *20*, 833–840.

Temoshok, L. (1987). Personality, coping style, emotion and cancer: Towards an integrative model. *Cancer Surveys*, *6*, 545–567.

Tennant, C., & Bebbington, P. (1978). The social causation of depression: A critique of the work of Brown and his colleagues. *Psychological Medicine*, *8*, 565–575.

Teshina, H. (1986). Recent biopsychosociological approaches to cancer study in Japan. In S.B. Day (Ed.), *Cancer, stress, and death* (pp. 79–87). New York: Plenum.

Thomas, P.D., Goodwin, J.M., & Goodwin, J.S. (1985). Effect of social support on stress-related changes in cholesterol level, uric acid level, and immune function in an elderly sample. *American Journal of Psychiatry*, *142*, 735–737.

Thurlbeck, W.M., Anderson, A.E., Jarvis, M., Mitchell, R.S., Pratt, P., Restrepo, G., Ryan, S.F., & Vincent, T. (1968). A co-operative study of certain measurements of emphysema. *Thorax*, *23*, 217–228.

Tomkins, S.S. (1968). A modified model of smoking behavior. In E.F. Borgatta & R. Evans (Eds.), *Smoking, health and behavior* (pp. 249–264). Chicago: Aldine.

Trichopolous, D. (1984). Passive smoking and lung cancer. *Lancet*, *2*, 684.

Trichopolous, D., Kalondidi, A., & Sparrow, L. (1983). Lung cancer and passive smoking: Conclusion of Greek study. *Lancet*, *2*, 677–678.

Trichopolous, D., Kalondidi, A., Sparrow, L., & Macmahon, B. (1981). Lung cancer and passive smoking. *International Journal of Cancer*, *27*, 1–4.

U.S. Department of Health and Human Services. (1988). *Nicotine addiction: A report of the Surgeon-General*. Rockville, MD: Office on Smoking & Health.

U.S. Surgeon General. (1979). *Health consequences of smoking*. Washington, DC: U.S. Department of Health and Human Services.

U.S. Surgeon General. (1982). *The health consequences of smoking—cancer*. Rockville, MD: U.S. Department of Health and Human Services.

U.S. Surgeon General. (1983). *Cardiovascular disease*. Rockville, MD: U.S. Department of Health and Human Services.

U.S. Surgeon General. (1986). *The health consequences of involuntary smoking*. Rockville, MD: U.S. Department of Health and Human Services.

U.S. Surgeon General. (1989). *Reducing the health consequences of smoking: 25 years of progress*. Rockville, MD: U.S. Department of Health and Human Services.

Vaillant, W.E., & Vaillant, C.O. (1990). Natural history of male psychological health: 12. A 45-year study of predictors of successful aging at age 65. *American Journal of Psychiatry*, *149*, 31–37.

Vecchia, C. la, Levi, F., & Gutzwiller, F. (1987). Fume et santé: Une épidemie évitable. *Medicine et Hygiene*, *45*, 3435–3462.

Wakefield, J. (1988). Results and methodological quality of smoking and health studies. *Personality & Individual Differences*, *9*, 465–477.

Waldron, H.A., & Vickerstaff, L. (1977). *Intimations of quality*. Oxford, UK: Nuffield Provincial Hospital Trust.

Walker, A.M. (1981). Proportion of disease attributable to the combined effect of two factors. *International Journal of Epidemiology*, *10*, 81–85.

Warburton, D.M. (1985). Addiction, dependence and habitual substance use. *Bulletin of the British Psychological Society*, *38*, 285–288.

Warburton, D.M. (1989). Is nicotine use an addiction? *The Psychologist*, *4*, 166–170.

Warburton, D.M., Revell, A., & Walter, A.C. (1988). Nicotine as a resource. In M.J. Rand & K. Tharan (Eds.), *The pharmacology of smoking* (pp. 359–373). Oxford, UK: IRL Press.

Wells, H.G. (1923). Relation of clinical to necropsy diagnosis in cancer and value of existing cancer statistics. *Journal of the American Medical Association*, *80*, 737–740.

Wilhelmsen, L., Berglund, G., Elmfeld, E., Tibblin, G., Wedel, H., Pennert, K., Vedin, A., Wilhelmsen, C., & Werker, L. (1986). The multifactor primary prevention trial in Goteborg. *European Heart Journal*, *7*, 279–288.

Wilhelmsen, L., Wedel, H., & Tibblin, G. (1973). Multivariate analysis of risk factors for coronary heart disease. *Circulation*, *48*, 950–958.

Willis, R.A. (1967). *Pathology of tumours* (4th ed.). London: Butterworth.

Wilson, E.B., & Burke, M.H. (1957). Some statistical observations as a cooperative study of human pulmonary pathology. *Proceedings of the National Academy of Sciences*, *43*, 1073–1078.

Wirsching, M., Stierlin, H., Weber, G., Wirsching, B., & Hoffman, F. (1981). Brustkrebs im Kontext: Ergebnisse einer Vorhersagestudie und Konsequenzen für die Therapie. *Zeitschrift für Psychosomatische Medizin, 27,* 239–252.

Workman, E.A., & La Via, M.F. (1987). T lymphocyte polyclonal proliferation and stress response style. *Psychological Reports, 60,* 1121–1122.

World Health Organization (Eds.). (1988). *A 5-year action plan: Smoke-free Europe.* Copenhagen: WHO Regional Office for Europe.

World Health Organization European Collaborative Group. (1982). Multifactorial trial in the prevention of coronary heart disease: 2. Risk factor change at two and four years. *European Heart Journal, 3,* 184–190.

Wynder, E.L. (1987). Workshop on guidelines to the epidemiology of weak association. *Preventive Medicine, 16,* 139–141.

Yerushalmy, J. (1966). On inferring causality from observed associations. In F.J. Ingelpinger, A.S. Relman, & M. Finland (Eds.), *Controversy in internal medicine* (pp. 68–75). London: W.B. Saunders.

Yesner, R., Selfman, N.A., & Feinstein, A.R. (1973). A reappraisal of histopathology in lung cancer and correlation of all types with antecedent cigarette smoking. *American Review of Respiratory Disease, 107,* 790–797.

Zonderman, A.B., Costa, P.T., & McCrae, R.R. (1989). Depression as a risk factor for cancer morbidity and mortally in a nationally representative sample. *Journal of the American Medical Association, 262,* 1191–1195.

Appendix:
Short Disease-Proneness Inventory

(For scoring, see instructions at end of inventory)

1. I find it very difficult to stand up for myself.   Yes   No
2. I have been complaining for years about various unfavorable conditions but am not able to change them.   Yes   No
3. I am mainly concerned with my own well-being.   Yes   No
4. I am usually content and happy with my daily activities.   Yes   No
5. I can express my feelings only when there are good reasons for them.   Yes   No
6. I don't believe in social rules and don't pay much attention to other people's expectations or the obligations I may have toward them.   Yes   No
7. I cannot live happily and contentedly with nor without a particular person.   Yes   No
8. I prefer to agree with others, rather than assert my own views.   Yes   No
9. Certain people are the most important causes of my personal misfortunes.   Yes   No
10. I alternate to a great degree between the positive and negative evaluation of people and conditions.   Yes   No
11. When I cannot achieve closeness with someone who is emotionally important to me, I have no difficulties in letting them go.   Yes   No
12. I have difficulties in showing my emotions because for every positive emotion there is a negative one.   Yes   No
13. My behavior toward other people alters from being very friendly and good-natured to being very hostile and aggressive.   Yes   No
14. I cannot life happily and contentedly in the presence or the absence of certain states or conditions; for example, I need my work but am unhappy doing it.   Yes   No
15. I tend to act more to fulfill the expectations of people close to me, rather than look after my own needs.   Yes   No

16. Certain conditions or situations are the most important
causes of my personal misfortunes.   Yes   No

17. With people I love, I keep changing from keeping them
at a great distance to stifling dependence, and from
stifling dependence to excessive distancing.   Yes   No

18. I can usually arrange things so that people who are
emotionally important to me are as close to or as distant
from me as I wish.   Yes   No

19. Reason, rather than emotion, guides my behavior.   Yes   No

20. I often expect others to fulfill agreements very strictly
but do not believe in doing so myself.   Yes   No

21. I often have thoughts that terrify me and make me
unhappy.   Yes   No

22. I tend to give in and abandon my own aims to achieve
harmony with other people.   Yes   No

23. I feel helpless against people or conditions that cause
great unhappiness for me, because I cannot change them.   Yes   No

24. When I am in a situation that I experience as
threatening, I immediately try to get other people to
help and support me.   Yes   No

25. When I fail to achieve my objectives, I can easily change
tack.   Yes   No

26. When people make emotional demands on me, I usually
react only rationally, never emotionally.   Yes   No

27. I usually act in a spontaneous manner, following my
immediate feelings without considering the actual
consequences.   Yes   No

28. Relations with certain people are always pretty
unsatisfactory, but there is nothing I can do about it.   Yes   No

29. I am unable to express my feelings and needs openly to
other people.   Yes   No

30. I always seem to be confronted with the undesirable
aspects of people and conditions.   Yes   No

31. When someone who is emotionally important to me
hurts me ever so slightly, I immediately dissociate
myself from that person.   Yes   No

32. I can manage to live fairly contentedly with or without
someone who is emotionally important to me.   Yes   No

33. I am quite unable to allow myself to be guided by
emotional considerations.   Yes   No

34. I often feel like attacking other people and crushing
them.   Yes   No

35. Certain situations and states (e.g., at my place of work)
tend to make me unhappy, but there is nothing I can do
to alter things.   Yes   No

36. I tend to accept conditions that work against my
    personal interests without being able to protest.   Yes   No
37. Certain people keep interfering with my personal
    development.   Yes   No
38. I expect others to live up to the highest moral standards
    but do not feel that these are binding on myself.   Yes   No
39. I can usually change my behavior to suit conditions.   Yes   No
40. My actions are never influenced by emotions to the
    degree that they might appear irrational.   Yes   No
41. When my partner demonstrates love toward me, I
    sometimes become particularly aggressive.   Yes   No
42. Certain bodily conditions (e.g., being overweight)
    make me unhappy, but I feel unable to do anything
    about it.   Yes   No
43. I often feel inhibited when it comes to openly showing
    negative feelings such as hatred, aggression, or anger.   Yes   No
44. Certain conditions keep interfering with my personal
    development.   Yes   No
45. I seek satisfaction of my own needs and desires first,
    regardless of the needs and rights of others.   Yes   No
46. I am usually capable of finding new points of view and
    successful, sometimes suprising, solutions for problems.   Yes   No
47. I always try to do what is rational and logically correct.   Yes   No
48. When I feel like attacking someone physically, I have no
    inhibitions about doing this at all.   Yes   No
49. I can relax bodily and mentally only very rarely; most of
    the time I am very tense.   Yes   No
50. I am inclined not to be demonstrative when emotional
    shocks upset me.   Yes   No
51. I cannot control excitement or stress in my life because
    this is dependent on the actions of other people.   Yes   No
52. When I make emotional demands on another person, I
    require immediate satisfaction.   Yes   No
53. I am independent in what I do and do not depend on
    other people when this works to my disadvantage.   Yes   No
54. I always try to express my needs and desires in a rational
    and reasonable manner.   Yes   No
55. I have no inhibitions in hurting myself physically if I feel
    like doing so.   Yes   No
56. I have great difficulties in entering into happy and
    contented relations with people.   Yes   No
57. When I feel emotionally let down I tend to be paralyzed
    and inhibited.   Yes   No
58. I cannot control excitement or stress in my life because
    this depends on conditions over which I have no control.   Yes   No

59. I usually find fulfillment in everyday situations that are *not* subject to ordinary rules, regulations, and expectations.   Yes No
60. When things don't work out, this does not make me give up but rather makes me change my way of doing things.   Yes No
61. I try to solve my problems in the light of relevant and rational consideration.   Yes No
62. I resent all moral obligations because they hamper and inhibit me.   Yes No
63. I am helpless when confronted with emotional shocks, depression, or anxiety.   Yes No
64. When something terrible happens to me, such as the death of a loved one, I am quite unable to express my emotions and desires.   Yes No
65. I can express my aims and desires clearly but feel that it is quite impossible to achieve them.   Yes No
66. As soon as someone becomes emotionally important for me, I tend to place contradictory demands on them, such as "Don't ever leave me" or "Get away from me."   Yes No
67. When things lead to harmful results for me, I have no trouble in changing my behavior to make for success.   Yes No
68. I only believe in things that can be proved scientifically and logically.   Yes No
69. When it benefits me, I have no hesitation in lying and pretending.   Yes No
70. I am seldom able to feel enthusiasm for anything.   Yes No

Scoring Instructions for
Short Disease-Proneness Inventory

Type 1: Add "Yes" answers to questions:
  1, 8, 15, 22, 29, 36, 43, 50, 57, 64
Type 2: Add "Yes" answers to questions:
  2, 9, 16, 23, 30, 37, 44, 51, 58, 65
Type 3: Add "Yes" answers to questions:
  3, 10, 17, 24, 31, 38, 45, 52, 59, 66
Type 4a: Add "Yes" answer to questions:
  4, 11, 18, 25, 32, 39, 46, 53, 60, 67
Type 4b: Add "No" answers to questions:
  7, 14, 21, 28, 35, 42, 49, 56, 63, 70
Type 5: Add "Yes" answers to questions:
  5, 12, 19, 26, 33, 40, 47, 54, 61, 68
Type 6: Add "Yes" answers to questions:
  6, 13, 20, 27, 34, 41, 48, 55, 62, 69

To decide type, add 4a and 4b, and divided by 2. A person's type is then the one on which he has the highest score. This is the ipsative way of scoring.

Another method is to take all 6 scores into account:

Type 1 is the cancer-prone type.
Type 2 is the coronary heart disease-type.
Type 3 is the alternating reaction type—reasonably healthy.
Type 4 is the autonomous, healthy type.
Type 5 is the rational-antiemotional type.
Type 6 is the antisocial, egocentric type.

(For further details, see Grossarth-Maticek, & Eysenck, 1990).

Author Index

Subject Index